SEXERCISE

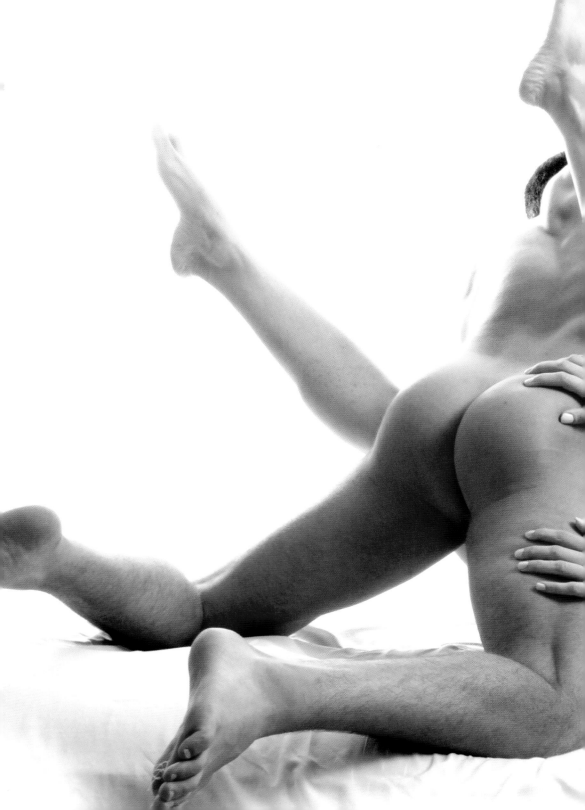

SEXERCISE

The Hottest Way to Burn Calories, Get a Better Body,
and Experience Mindblowing Orgasms

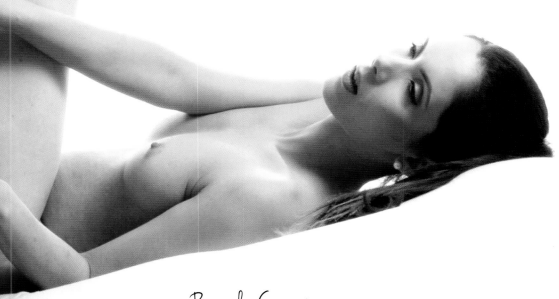

Beverly Cummings

QUIVER

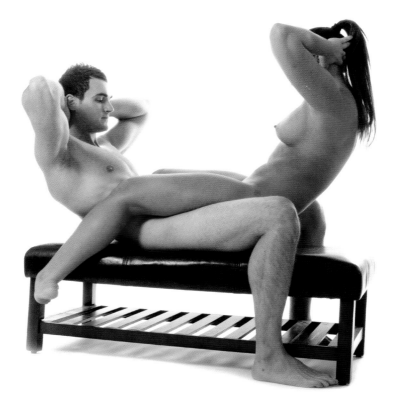

Compilation © 2013 Quiver
Photography © 2013 Moseley Road, Inc.

This 2013 edition published by
Quiver, a member of
Quayside Publishing Group
100 Cummings Center
Suite 406-L
Beverly, MA 01915-6101
www.quiverbooks.com

Produced for Quayside Publishing Group by
Moseley Road Inc.
123 Main Street
Irvington, NY 10533

Photography by JPC

16 15 14 13 12   1 2 3 4 5

ISBN 978-1-59233-554-1

Printed in Singapore

CONTENTS

INTRODUCTION

All sex provides some form of exercise, whether it's little more than a gentle stretch of the inner thigh muscles for her with a quick blast of the glutes and hip-flexor muscles for him or, preferably, a full aerobic marathon for both partners that leaves them in an exhausted, sweaty heap having burned up a couple of thousand calories apiece. In recent years, sex and fitness enthusiasts like myself have started taking this idea a little further and have come up with a whole host of "sexercises" that focus on honing and toning specific body parts. Sexercise is just like traditional exercise except that instead of working out at the gym, you're making out in the bedroom; and instead of using the resistance of weights, you're resisting the irresistible force of your lover's gorgeous body. It's like traditional resistance training, but it's a heck of a lot more fun.

Why Sexercise?

The benefits are boundless, a virtuous cycle of improved health coupled with an ever more exciting sex life. The more sexercise you do, the fitter you get; the fitter you get, the more you get out of the sexercise. OK, so a quick flip through the pages will have some of you thinking, "never in a million years would I be able to do that!" You may be right, but there are plenty of sexercises for everybody at every level. If you stick with it, you'll soon be able to complete some of those sexercises you considered impossible at first glance. You might find that with a long-term partner, sexercise will rekindle fading passions and get you trying a lot of new things. You'll find yourself laughing as you try moves for the first time. Some might think that sex and laughter are incompatible, but I disagree wholeheartedly—yes, sex can be steamy and passionate, but it can and should be fun. Laughter, along with exercise and sex, is one of the all-time great stress busters, and that's no small advantage in our modern society.

Gymnastics Without the Gym

All you need to get started is a willing partner and a private space—there's absolutely no special equipment required. The bedroom is a natural option for the private space but by no means the only one; you can perform most of these sexercises just as easily in the living room as long as you're sure you won't be disturbed. The sexercises themselves involve highly erotic and sometimes challenging positions that combine steamy sex with strength, stamina, and flexibility work for every major muscle group. For those more interested in the sex than the exercise (so, about ninety-nine percent of us), there are plenty of positions that are just begging for the introduction of sex toys. Generally, I've left that to your own imagination.

Again, some of the sexercises have elements of either male or female domination or submission and, being an avid fan of a little gentle bondage-play myself, I have sometimes pointed out positions where a submissive man or woman might feel especially aroused or where a soft spank or two would not go amiss. Needless to say, such sex play should only ever be indulged in with the consent of your partner.

Your Sexercise Schedule

For the most part, I've divided the book into sections based on major body parts but the first chapter introduces some "steamy stretches" because a little gentle stretching is the first thing you should do to warm up before any strenuous exercise. And, as you'll see, the warm up doesn't have to be dull!

How often should you sexercise? I have suggested workouts with appropriate schedules at the end of each chapter, focusing on the abdominals, say, and perhaps having a common theme, such as all being in a standing position or all being especially arousing to women who like a little bondage play—oops, there I go again. However, feel free to mix and match the sexercises as you see fit, and to fit in with your own sexual preferences. What I would say, however, is don't attempt anything that you're not one hundred percent sure you—

and, of course, your partner—are capable of performing. Some of the more challenging sexercises need great strength or agility just to get into the position in the first place and these should be left until you have sufficiently improved your own fitness or are perhaps best left to the lucky superfit few.

Love Muscles

The final chapter covers cardiovascular sexercise. OK, the heart is actually an organ composed of muscle tissue and other stuff, but it is vital to great sex as it gets his other love muscle (which, yes I know, is also an organ) pumped up and ready for action, and once you start your own pumping from the hips, your cardiovascular system helps to keep you going...and going...and, eventually anyway, coming.

And let's face it, there's not much point in having strong abdominals if they're hidden beneath a layer of fat—as well as pumping

up those muscles you need to get the blood pumping through your heart to help raise your metabolism and burn the maximum amount of calories. Translated into sexual terms, this is only good news as it means you finally get to let go and do what feels most natural—going at a full gallop until you both collapse into that exhausted, sweaty heap I mentioned earlier. Anyway, the best way to learn this stuff is on the job. Let's get busy.

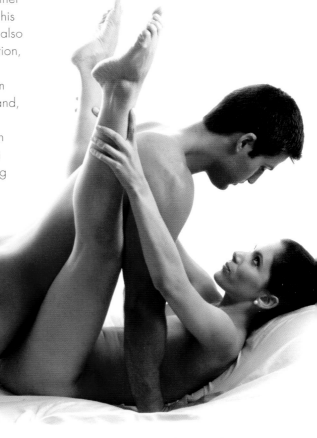

ANATOMY

One thing I hear from sexercise initiates again and again is, "I'm using muscles I didn't know I had." That's another great benefit: You really—I mean really—get to know your own and your partner's body inside out. And though that may sound daunting to some, it's actually immensely liberating. I've included these anatomical diagrams so that you can familiarize yourself with the specific muscle groups being trained—those areas where you are likely to feel the "burn" when you perform the exercise correctly. That burn is the holy grail of every fitness enthusiast as it means you are working that muscle and strengthening and toning it.

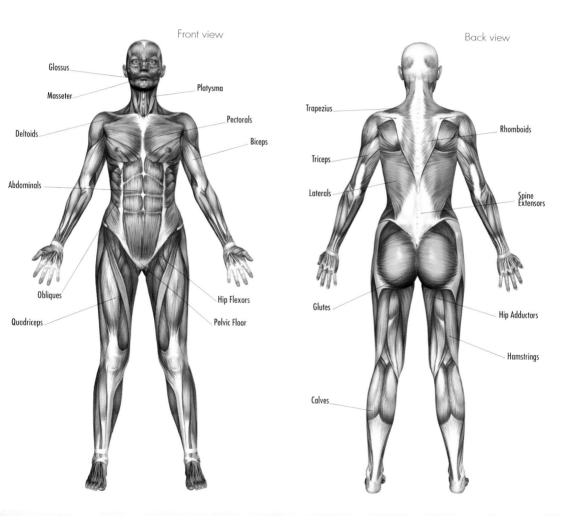

Front view

Glossus
Masseter
Platysma
Pectorals
Deltoids
Biceps
Abdominals
Obliques
Hip Flexors
Quadriceps
Pelvic Floor

Back view

Trapezius
Rhomboids
Triceps
Laterals
Spine Extensors
Glutes
Hip Adductors
Hamstrings
Calves

STEAMY STRETCHES

Stretching before sexercise should be the equivalent of foreplay before sex—neglect it at your peril. As well as warming up the muscles and getting the blood pumping a little faster, it should be a sexually arousing experience and a taster of things to come. My advice is not to get naked straightaway but, instead, wear the shorts and T-shirt that you would wear for normal exercise, or skimpy lingerie if you prefer. These stretches are designed so that you can work together, not just because assisted stretches are more effective than stretching alone, but also because watching your partner is arousing and the contact with your partner's body, even clothed, builds up a sense of excitement and anticipation. The physical signs of your arousal will very soon be evident, but resist the urge to strip until you have finished the stretching workout—anticipation is everything.

THE SPLIT SWITCH

A superb stretch for the oft-neglected inner thighs, as well as the hips, hamstrings, and back. It's a great starting point because you're holding hands and you can explore your partner's body with your eyes but cannot caress at this stage. That's a good thing; we all know that the brain is our most powerful sex organ and, anticipating what lies ahead, it will soon be activating those pleasure hormones.

HOT TIP

Ladies, as he pulls you toward him he'll have a great view of your breasts and won't fail to notice your nipples swell beneath your t-shirt. You, in turn, will notice the increasing bulge in his shorts. Make no secret of your relish and stare greedily, telling him how much you want him inside you and what you want him to do to you. Guys, same goes for you, tell her how great she looks and how turned-on you are. Remember, this is sexercise—sex definitely comes first.

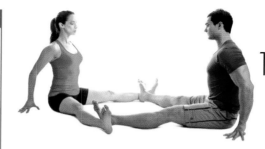

1 The woman sits upright on the floor with her legs spread as widely as is comfortable and her toes pointing upward. The man adopts a similar position opposite her and places the soles of his feet just above her inner ankles.

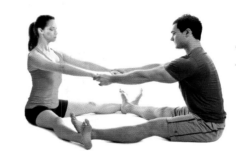

2 The lovers grasp each other's hands, keeping the back as flat as possible with the abdomen muscles contracted, the chest elevated, and their necks extended upward.

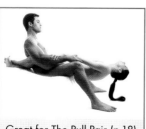

Great for The Pull Pair (p.18)

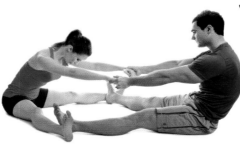

3 The man then gently leans backward, pulling his partner forward. Hold for thirty seconds then relax and repeat the process. Then switch roles and repeat the entire exercise for two sets.

ASSISTED CHEST STRETCH

This is an excellent stretch for the chest and shoulders. Keep talking, telling your partner when the stretch is sufficiently strong and taking care that he or she is relaxed and comfortable. Her beautiful breasts (or his powerful pecs) are clearly the focus of attention here. In between sets, take the opportunity to caress her breasts through her T-shirt while she leans back to receive a passionate kiss.

HOT TIP

While you are in this seated position you can also focus on those all-important inner-thigh and pelvic-floor muscles. Ask him to move around to the front and place his hands on your inner thighs to assist the stretch. Similarly, you can encourage him with his pelvic-floor exercise by lightly cupping his testicles to feel them lift slightly when he contracts the correct muscles.

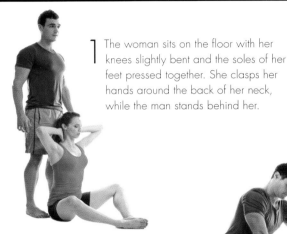

1 The woman sits on the floor with her knees slightly bent and the soles of her feet pressed together. She clasps her hands around the back of her neck, while the man stands behind her.

2 The man then bends his legs and gently places his knees against the sides of her middle back. He then reaches down and rests his forearms across her elbows.

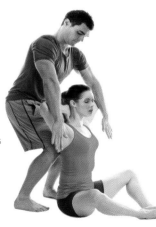

3 The man then gently presses her elbows toward his hips, while she resists the pressure with her arms. Hold for ten seconds, then relax and repeat the process. Switch roles and repeat the entire exercise for two sets.

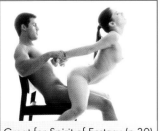

Great for Spirit of Ecstasy (p.30)

ASSISTED SPINAL EXTENSION

Once again, this works on the inner thighs, but it actually focuses more on the abdominals and the spine extensors—long muscles stretching from the butt to the shoulders that are crucial to good posture and core stability. Whoever is assisting the stretch enjoys a great view of his or her partner's sexy buns. Why resist the urge to have a gentle squeeze or two?

HOT TIP

When relaxing between sets, kneel back up into the starting position and, requesting (or demanding) that your partner steps around to stand before you, gently nibble the shaft of his penis through his shorts to really start hotting things up.

1 The woman kneels with her buttocks resting lightly on her heels. She then opens her knees slightly and engages her abdominal muscles.

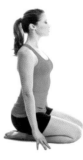
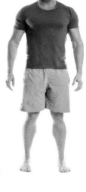

2 She stretches her arms forward to rest her forearms and palms flat on the floor. The man places his hands on her outer thighs. As she stretches her arms and chest forward and down, he applies a gentle downward pressure to her thighs.

3 Hold the stretch for thirty seconds then relax and return to the starting position. Repeat for a second set, then switch roles and perform the entire sequence once again.

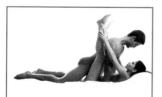

Great for Do the Lotion Motion (p.134)

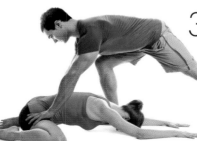

ASSISTED PRETZEL

Great for the glutes and thighs, this stretch also works the hip flexors, abdominals, shoulders, and chest. It will prepare the woman's legs and hips for some high-rise action as in the Upstairs, Downstairs sexercise (see p.24). Meanwhile, it also stretches her obliques, ready for such moves as the Twisted Sister (see p.62). And remember guys, her thighs are highly-charged erogenous zones, so be sure to take time out to caress and kiss them between sets.

HOT TIP

Some of the sexercises in this book require the man to adopt submissive sexual postures with his legs raised, such as the Erotic Aerobic sexercise (see p.124), so guys need to work hard on this stretch too—especially those who get a kick out of being dominated sexually.

1 The woman lies on her back with her left leg fully extended and her right leg bent with the sole of her foot flat on the floor. The man kneels to her right.

2 The woman then raises her hips off the floor and, tilting her torso approximately three inches to her left, she crosses her bent leg over the extended one.

3 The man places his left hand on the woman's shoulder and gently presses his other hand down on her right thigh. Hold for thirty seconds then repeat with the opposite leg. Switch roles and perform the whole sequence again.

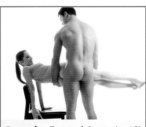

Great for Twisted Sister (p.62)

HAPPY BABY

Once again, we're working on the glutes, hip-flexors, and thighs, but this is also an excellent stretch for the lower back. I find it's best to start with the guy stretching first. When it comes to the woman's turn, it's impossible to resist doing some fancy footwork when her feet are so close to his groin. Her digital dexterity will inevitably bring the stretching session—and general foreplay—to a close; it's time for some serious penetrative sexercise.

HOT TIP

Once she has massaged his penis with her feet for a couple of minutes, it's time for him to reciprocate and get the real action started. The man should take this opportunity to kneel before her, remove her shorts, and pleasure her orally. There's no going back from here.

1 The woman lies on her back with both legs extended and her arms held away from her torso with her palms facing upward. The man stands over her with a foot placed on either side of her waist.

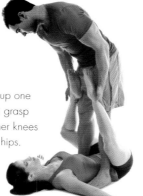

2 The woman then raises her legs up one at a time so that her partner can grasp each ankle. She slightly bends her knees and turns out both legs from the hips.

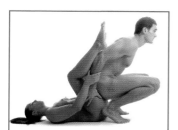

Great for Bumping Rumps (p.86)

3 The man then brings his partner's ankles to the front of his body, holding them against the top of his thighs. Hold the stretch for thirty seconds then relax and repeat for a second set. Switch roles and perform the entire sequence for two sets.

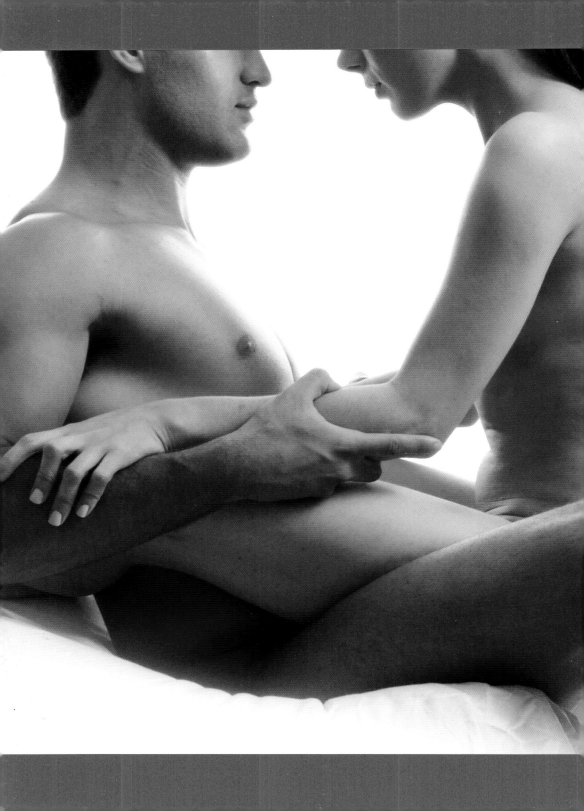

AMOROUS ARMS

Guys and their "guns"; there's nothing that needs to be said about how important arms are to a man. Even if a man is strictly a missionary-position-only guy—as, alas, too many still are—he will still need strong arms to support himself until that missionary is accomplished. Many of the positions in this book require a man to have powerful arms just to get into the position in the first place. And, let's face it, few things make a woman feel better than that "light-as-a-feather" feeling as her man picks her up effortlessly—or at least without putting his back out. Ladies, too, are becoming more and more appreciative of the beauty of sleek, strong arms on the female form, and the sexercises in this chapter will help her to gain and maintain great arms that mean she can indeed wear that sexy, sleeveless dress, and which will also serve her well for some sensational sex.

THE PULL PAIR

As well as being a great workout for the arms, the Pull Pair really works on those abdominal muscles and it's usually the abs burn that draws play to a close. As with all these sexercises, start out gently, leaning back just a little way in the first sessions and building up over time. This is a fun face-to-face sexercise, so take advantage and reward yourselves after each successful set of ten reps by giving those jaw muscles a workout with some serious necking.

MAJOR TARGETS

Deltoids	Deltoids
Triceps	Triceps
Abdominals	Abdominals

HOT TIP

Penetration is deep and this sexercise also provides a great opportunity for the woman to work on her pelvic-floor muscles, gripping his penis as she leans back and releasing the delicious pressure as she rises slowly up, allowing him to fully penetrate once again before he takes his turn to lean.

1 The man situates himself as far as possible from the edge of the bed while keeping the soles of his feet in contact with the floor for stability. The woman then sits in his lap—facing toward her lover—and wraps her legs around his lower back.

2 The lovers grasp each other's forearms in a Roman handshake then, while the man leans his torso back slightly to support his partner's weight, the woman reclines slowly over the edge of the bed, keeping her stomach muscles tense and feeling the stretch in her shoulders and triceps.

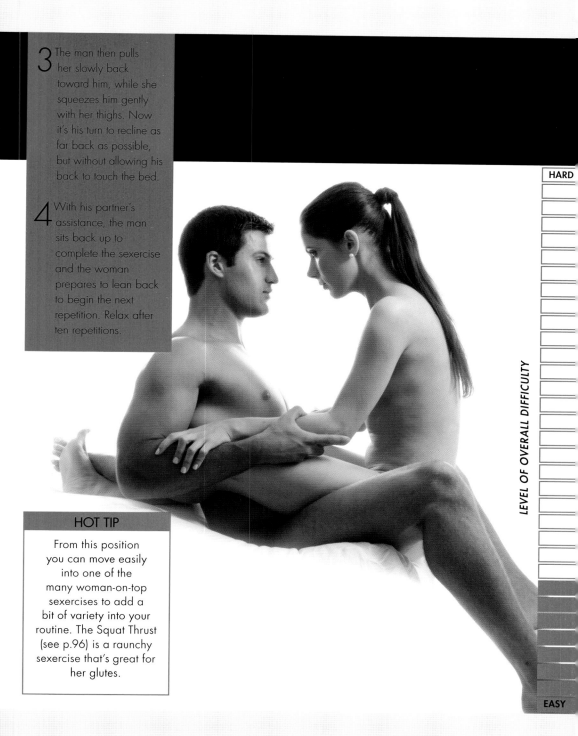

3 The man then pulls her slowly back toward him, while she squeezes him gently with her thighs. Now it's his turn to recline as far back as possible, but without allowing his back to touch the bed.

4 With his partner's assistance, the man sits back up to complete the sexercise and the woman prepares to lean back to begin the next repetition. Relax after ten repetitions.

HOT TIP

From this position you can move easily into one of the many woman-on-top sexercises to add a bit of variety into your routine. The Squat Thrust (see p.96) is a raunchy sexercise that's great for her glutes.

HARD

LEVEL OF OVERALL DIFFICULTY

EASY

THE DIVE BOMBER

The Dive Bomber is a great upper-body and arm workout for the man but is more of a leg workout for the woman. It can be difficult at first to coordinate all that bumping and grinding with the shoulder raises, so be sure to try it moving slowly for the first few sessions. Although some fitness fanatics have been known to employ dumbbells for this sexercise, it's not recommended—you don't want to take "knockout sex" too literally.

MAJOR TARGETS

Deltoids	Hamstrings
Laterals	Quadriceps
Pectorals	Glutes

HOT TIP

For the woman, this is a great opportunity to fondle her partner's gorgeous, muscular rump. Try introducing a little playful spanking to liven things up (with your lover's permission of course).

1 The woman lies back on the bed with her legs raised and open, keeping them as straight as she can without discomfort. Her partner enters her from the side of the bed, extending his right arm straight down to support his weight.

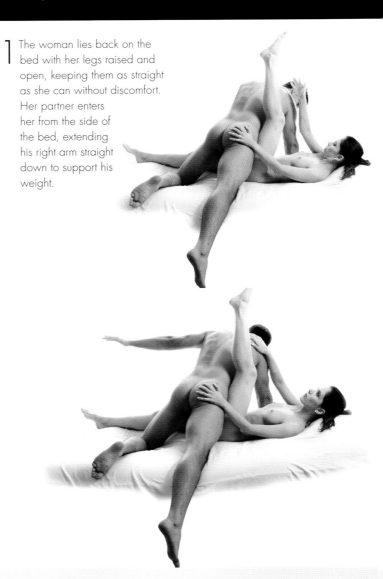

2 The man then raises his left arm and holds it at shoulder height for approximately a minute.

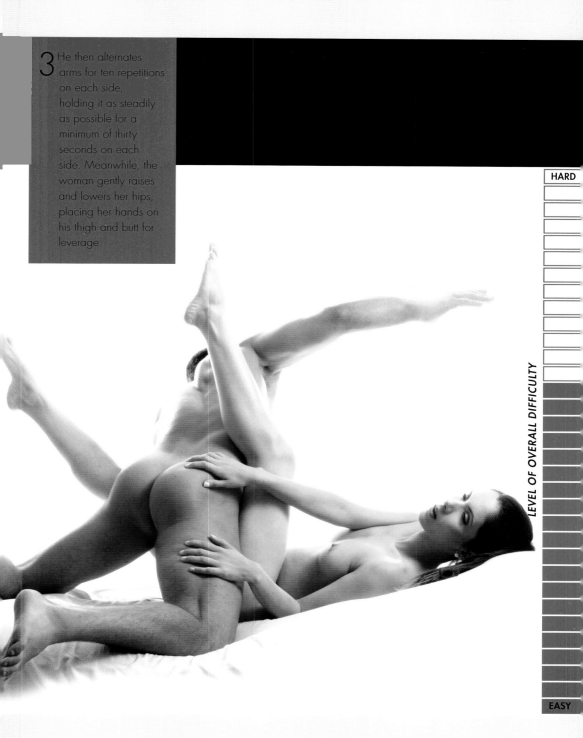

3 He then alternates arms for ten repetitions on each side, holding it as steadily as possible for a minimum of thirty seconds on each side. Meanwhile, the woman gently raises and lowers her hips, placing her hands on his thigh and butt for leverage.

HARD

LEVEL OF OVERALL DIFFICULTY

EASY

A MATTER OF THRUST

As his arms work to keep her elevated, her arms are also working to counteract his thrusts—even when she is just supporting her weight on her forearms. She can raise her game further by introducing a few declined push-ups, making this a fabulous full-body workout. He works on his legs, too, by bending them slightly each time she lowers her chest to the floor —helping her, and helping himself to a great view of her butt.

MAJOR TARGETS

♂	♀
Triceps	Deltoids
Deltoids	Triceps
Trapezius	Pectorals

HOT TIP

If the woman is superfit you might decide to take her on a tour of the room, with her "walking" hand over hand while you follow along behind focusing on trying to stay "plugged in"— playing "wheelbarrows" was great fun as a kid, right? Well it's a lot more fun now.

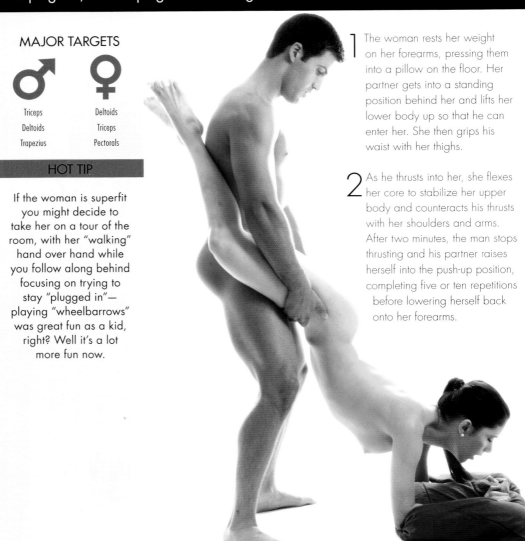

1 The woman rests her weight on her forearms, pressing them into a pillow on the floor. Her partner gets into a standing position behind her and lifts her lower body up so that he can enter her. She then grips his waist with her thighs.

2 As he thrusts into her, she flexes her core to stabilize her upper body and counteracts his thrusts with her shoulders and arms. After two minutes, the man stops thrusting and his partner raises herself into the push-up position, completing five or ten repetitions before lowering herself back onto her forearms.

3 He helps his partner at this stage by bending his legs slightly as she lowers her chest to the floor, working his glutes and hamstrings. Try to keep going for ten minutes, with the man alternating between thrusting and squatting, while she alternates between leaning on her forearms and brief push-up stages.

HOT TIP

Perhaps the most difficult thing about this position is getting into it in the first place. You might find it easier to start off with the man sitting on a chair. She straddles his lap facing in the same direction and then leans forward to take her weight on her hands. He then stands up carefully and she lowers herself onto her forearms and clasps her legs around his waist.

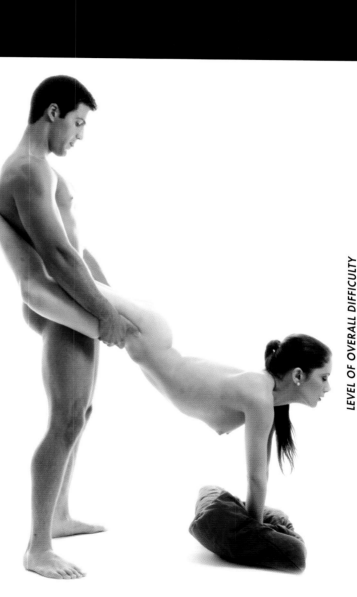

HARD

LEVEL OF OVERALL DIFFICULTY

EASY

UPSTAIRS, DOWNSTAIRS

The Upstairs, Downstairs sexercise is a great workout for her shoulders and chest, while he gets to work on his biceps. By squatting to support her weight he also gets to work his glutes and hamstrings. The intense sexual pleasure here is heightened for both partners as the woman raises and lowers her leg to subtly vary the angle of entry.

MAJOR TARGETS

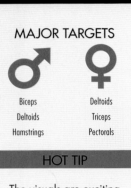

Biceps	Deltoids
Deltoids	Triceps
Hamstrings	Pectorals

HOT TIP

The visuals are exciting here as he has an unrestricted view of her face and exquisite breasts. She can watch his face and witness his excitement but also his frustration as he is unable to reach down and touch her. She can relieve this frustration by momentarily lowering her raised leg and wrapping both around his waist so that she supports herself while he reaches down to touch her.

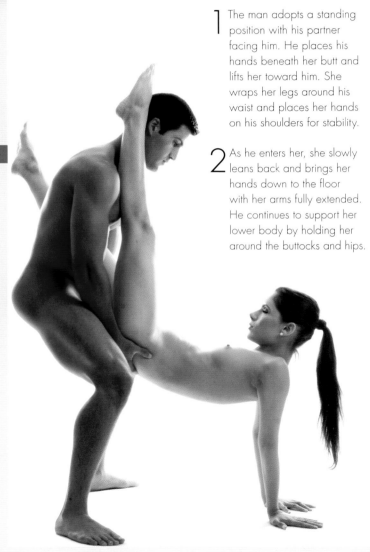

1 The man adopts a standing position with his partner facing him. He places his hands beneath her butt and lifts her toward him. She wraps her legs around his waist and places her hands on his shoulders for stability.

2 As he enters her, she slowly leans back and brings her hands down to the floor with her arms fully extended. He continues to support her lower body by holding her around the buttocks and hips.

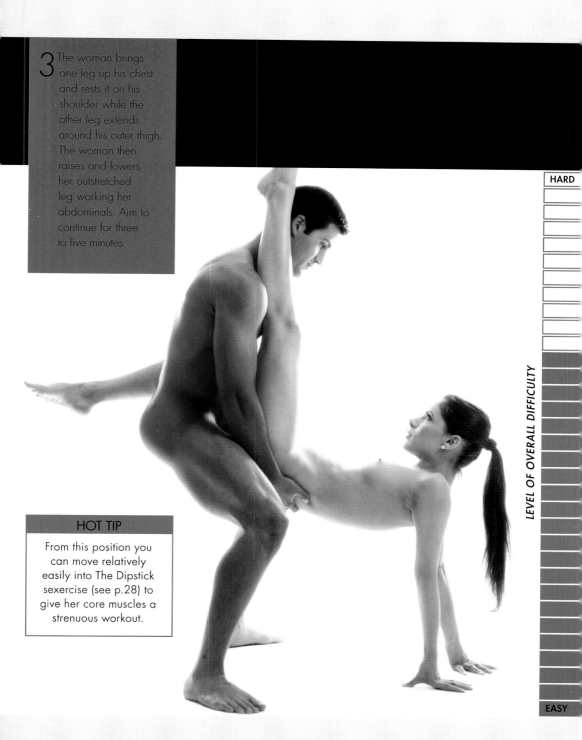

3 The woman brings one leg up his chest and rests it on his shoulder while the other leg extends around his outer thigh. The woman then raises and lowers her outstretched leg working her abdominals. Aim to continue for three to five minutes.

HOT TIP

From this position you can move relatively easily into The Dipstick sexercise (see p.28) to give her core muscles a strenuous workout.

HARD

LEVEL OF OVERALL DIFFICULTY

EASY

THE PLOW

The Plow is a supreme workout for her shoulders and entire upper body. Meanwhile, the man gets to work his shoulders and triceps by raising and lowering her hips. Of course, as any farmer will tell you, one of the joys of plowing is the wonderful view—in this case the man gets to admire her beautiful butt as he merrily plows her furrow; she is stuck with an extreme close-up of the chair back.

MAJOR TARGETS

Deltoids	Deltoids
Triceps	Triceps
Hamstrings	Pectorals

HOT TIP

You can vary this sexercise by adding a few squat sets into the mix. You know the routine—bend the knees, keeping them behind the toes, and keep the torso upright and contracted. Press into your heels to stand back up. By shifting the angle of incline, she will be shifting the work from her upper pectorals to her lower pectorals.

1 The woman adopts a kneeling position and rests her forearms against the seat of a chair or the side of a bed.

2 Approaching from behind, her lover lifts her from the hips and enters her as she locks her legs around his lower back.

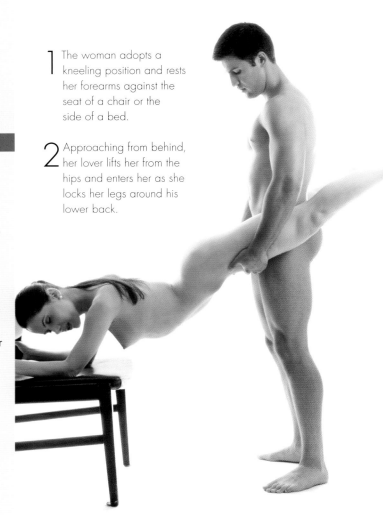

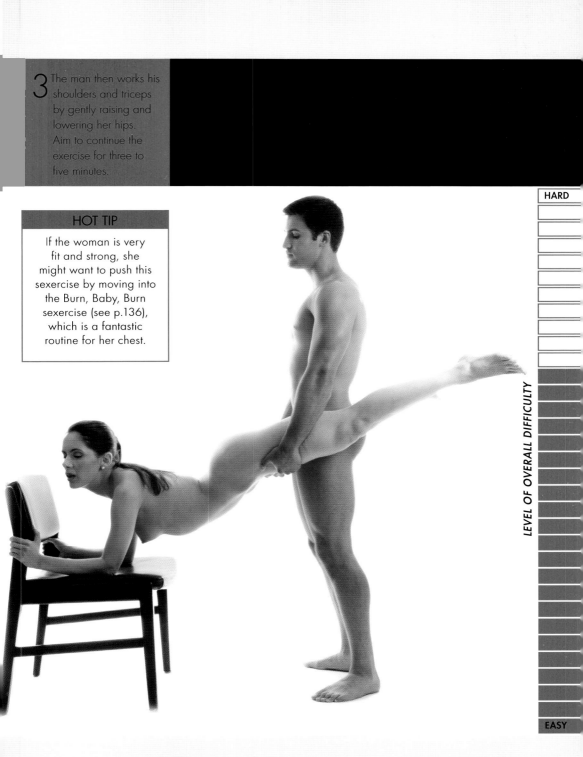

3 The man then works his shoulders and triceps by gently raising and lowering her hips. Aim to continue the exercise for three to five minutes.

HOT TIP

If the woman is very fit and strong, she might want to push this sexercise by moving into the Burn, Baby, Burn sexercise (see p.136), which is a fantastic routine for her chest.

HARD

LEVEL OF OVERALL DIFFICULTY

EASY

THE DIPSTICK

The Dipstick is an inverted position that, for the woman at least, delivers all the substantial benefits of a headstand: Strengthening the core, stimulating the brain, and nourishing the face by increasing the circulation to the skin of the cheeks and forehead. It's also a great workout for the trapezius and deltoid muscles. For him, this is an all-round arm workout—the challenge will be keeping his stick dipped because of the extreme angle of entry.

MAJOR TARGETS

Deltoids	Deltoids
Triceps	Trapezius
Hamstrings	Pectorals

HOT TIP

The extreme angle of entry, although hard to maintain, creates a delicious pressure on the head of his penis and the anterior wall of her vagina—home to the legendary G-spot.

1 The man stands in front of his partner and places his hands beneath her butt to lift her toward him. He enters her as she wraps her legs around his waist and her arms around his shoulders.

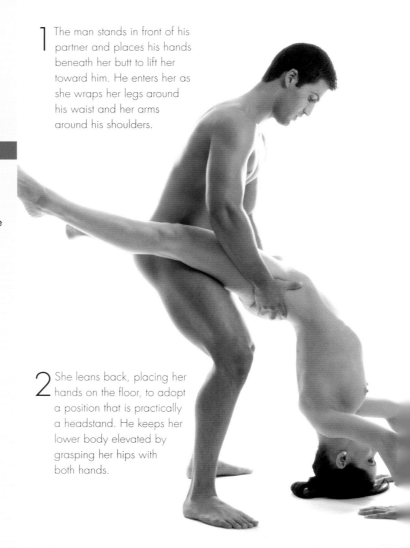

2 She leans back, placing her hands on the floor, to adopt a position that is practically a headstand. He keeps her lower body elevated by grasping her hips with both hands.

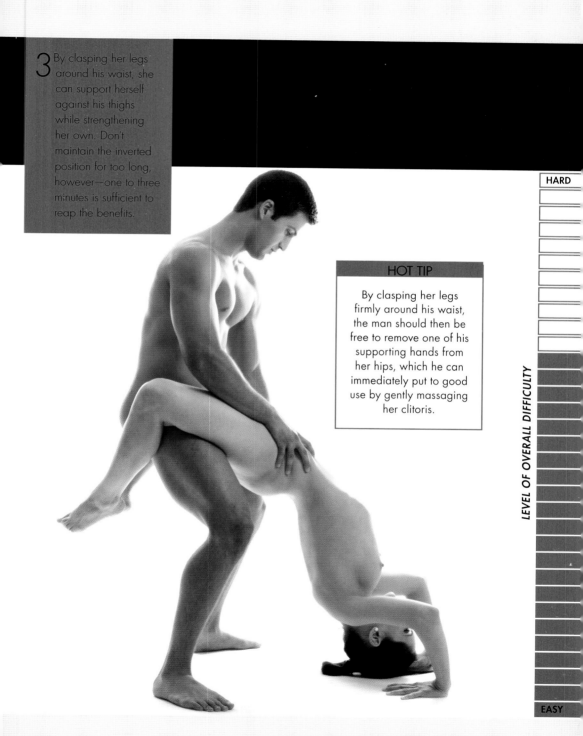

3 By clasping her legs around his waist, she can support herself against his thighs while strengthening her own. Don't maintain the inverted position for too long, however—one to three minutes is sufficient to reap the benefits.

HOT TIP

By clasping her legs firmly around his waist, the man should then be free to remove one of his supporting hands from her hips, which he can immediately put to good use by gently massaging her clitoris.

LEVEL OF OVERALL DIFFICULTY

HARD

EASY

SPIRIT OF ECSTASY

A great workout for the man's upper back and shoulders, as well as his arms, Spirit of Ecstasy is equally effective for strengthening the woman's entire upper body. Sexually, it provides a great opportunity for him to butt-gaze, while she wriggles her hips to ensure maximum penetration and struggles against the constant urge to sing the theme song from the blockbuster movie *Titanic*.

MAJOR TARGETS

Biceps	Deltoids
Rhomboids	Rhomboids
Pectorals	Pectorals

HOT TIP

By flexing her feet against the floor the woman is also able to work her legs, making this a great workout for her entire body. The man is limited in his ability to move, so the woman takes control by maneuvering her hips to continually adjust of the angle and depth of penetration.

1 The man sits on a chair with a back that is sufficiently narrow to allow him to move his elbows back. His feet should be flat on the floor in front of him. The woman sits in his lap with her back toward him and he enters her.

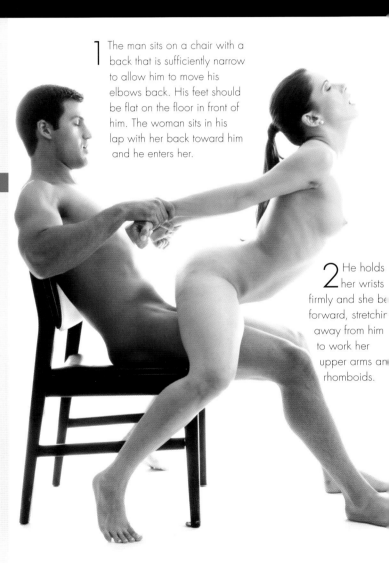

2 He holds her wrists firmly and she be forward, stretchir away from him to work her upper arms an rhomboids.

3 Keeping his elbows bent and working from the shoulders, the man then gently pulls his lover back toward him. Continue the movement for at least twenty repetitions.

HOT TIP

Guys, if you've ever looked longingly at a Rolls-Royce Silver Shadow and wondered what it would be like to bang the exquisite little creature—known as "the Spirit of Ecstasy"—that adorns the hood, you should call a psychiatrist immediately. However, if your shrink is unable to help, this sexercise is the nearest you'll get to fulfilling your messed-up fantasy.

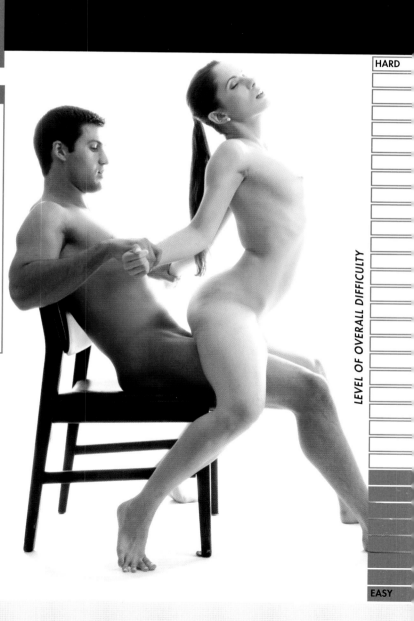

HARD

LEVEL OF OVERALL DIFFICULTY

EASY

ARMS WORKOUT 1

This stand-up/hang down workout combines four sexercises that will help you to develop sleek, strong, muscular arms, and avoid that flabby underarm excess know as "bingo wings."

UPSTAIRS, DOWNSTAIRS
(pages 24–25)

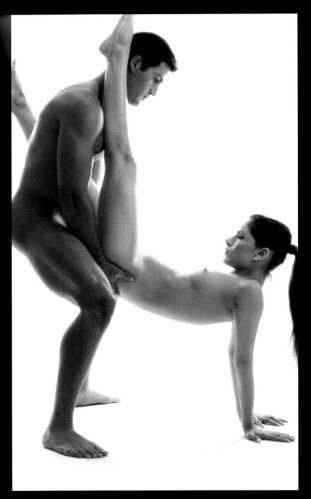

THE DIPSTICK
(pages 28–29)

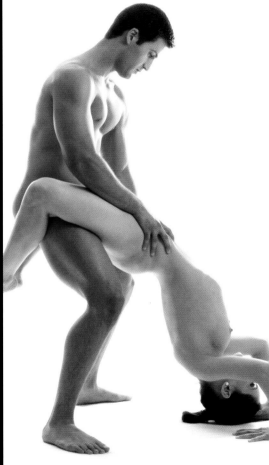

DURATION
Perform each position for
2 minutes minimum, increasing 30
seconds per additional workout

SCHEDULE
Once every other week

A MATTER OF THRUST
(pages 22–23)

THE PLOW
(pages 30–31)

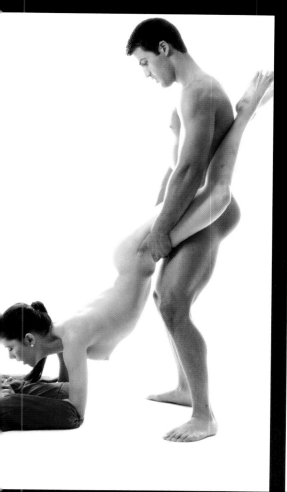

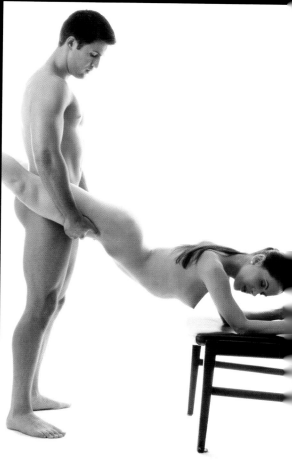

ARMS WORKOUT 2

Here are four more sexercises that will enable you to build up beautiful biceps and triceps while enjoying a varied range of positions and, consequently, a varied range of entry angles.

THE PULL PAIR
(pages 18–19)

SPIRIT OF ECSTASY
(pages 30–31)

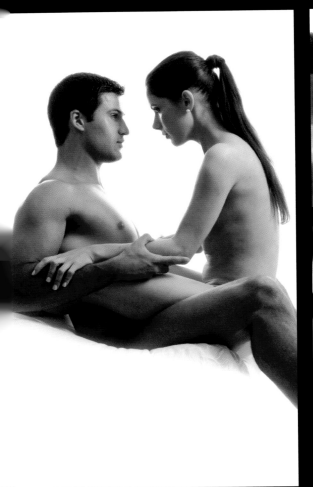

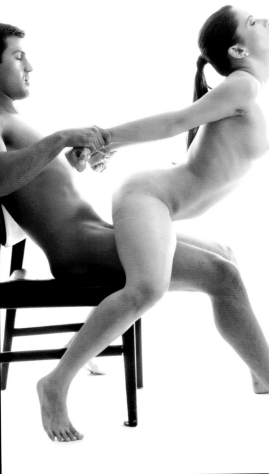

DURATION
Perform each position for
2 minutes minimum, increasing 30
seconds per additional workout

SCHEDULE
Once every other week

THE DIVE BOMBER
(pages 20–21)

BURN, BABY, BURN
(pages 136–37)

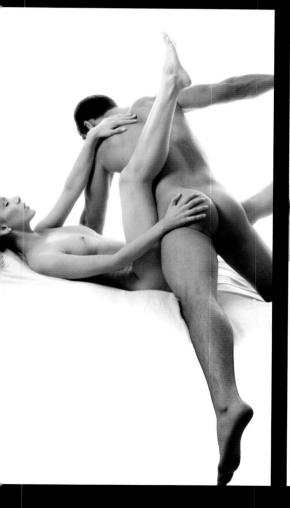

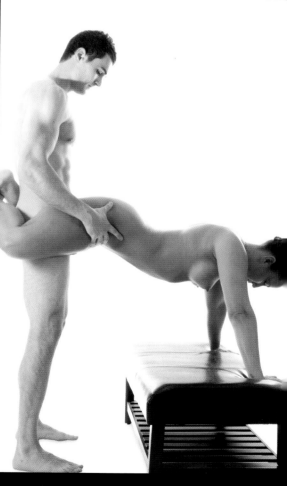

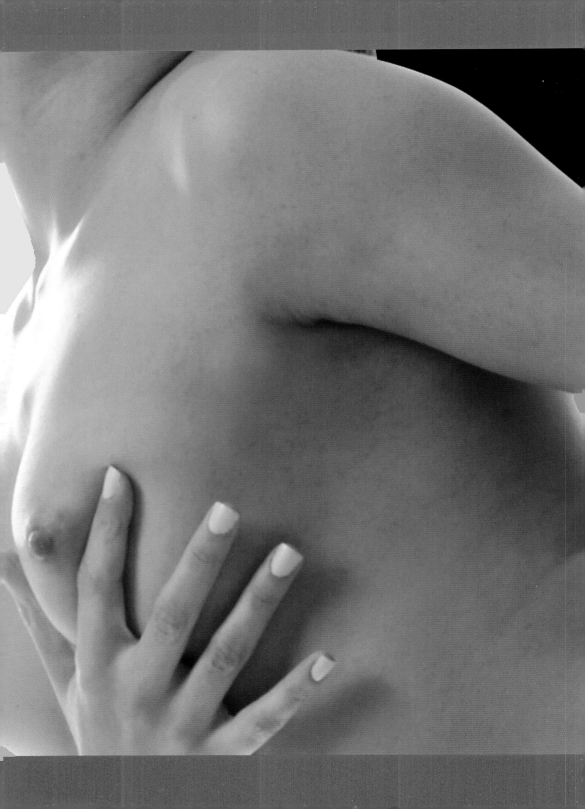

BEST CHEST

A woman's breasts are among her most powerful sexual assets and are a potent symbol of femininity. Although the breasts themselves don't contain any muscle mass, the pectoral muscles in the chest that help to support them need to be kept strong to help your breasts stay firm and inviting. Similarly, women often cite a guy's chest as his most attractive body part. From a woman's viewpoint his powerful pecs contrast with her curvy softness to make her feel feminine and protected. All of the sexercises in this section will help to strengthen and tone your pectorals. Many of the sexercises also work the back, however. Why? Because the back and shoulder muscles work to stabilize the pectorals. They are vital for good posture and, ladies, you already know that if you improve your body posture your breasts instantly appear higher and firmer.

OPEN FOR BUSINESS

As well as being a great workout for the chest—focusing particularly on the larger pectoralis major for him and the smaller but equally important pectoralis minor for her—this sexercise also works on those back and ab muscles. It's very stimulating for the male as he feels, and is, very much the dominant partner in this position. However, for her, it's impossible to maintain this position for too long.

MAJOR TARGETS

Pectorals	Pectorals
Deltoids	Rhomboids
Biceps	Abdominals

HOT TIP

This is an exciting position for a physically fit woman who likes to introduce a little bondage into her sex play. She feels deliciously vulnerable and her movements are very much restricted by her lover's grip. Also, the further your faces are apart the more impersonal sex feels, and this feeling is intensified by the fact that she is facing away from him.

1 This chest extension begins with the woman mounting her partner from a sitting position facing outward. The man holds her firmly by the forearms and stands up, while she keeps her body at a right angle to his.

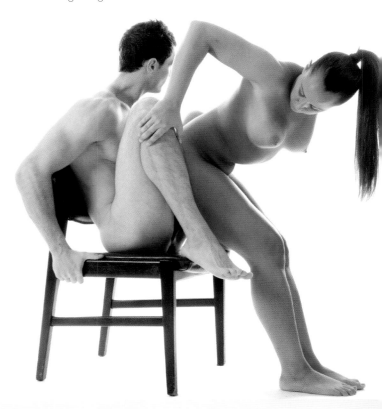

2 The man brings his shoulder blades back to open his chest while the woman wraps her thighs around his waist. Try to hold the position for one to two minutes.

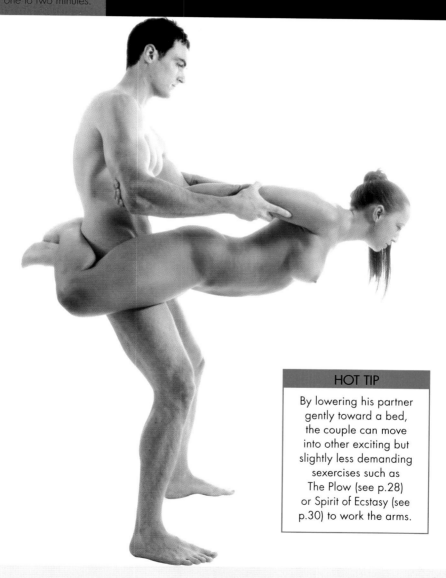

HARD

LEVEL OF OVERALL DIFFICULTY

EASY

HOT TIP

By lowering his partner gently toward a bed, the couple can move into other exciting but slightly less demanding sexercises such as The Plow (see p.28) or Spirit of Ecstasy (see p.30) to work the arms.

THE DOUBLE UP

The Double Up is effectively a modified push-up and, as such, is a wonderful workout for the chest and arms. The woman gently stretches her torso upward from a prone position while her partner adopts a similar posture facing in the opposite direction. The extreme angle of entry can make it difficult to keep the penis from slipping out, so only very gentle movement of the hips is advisable.

MAJOR TARGETS

Pectorals	Pectorals
Triceps	Triceps
Deltoids	Deltoids

HOT TIP

By fully extending her arms and creating an arch in her back from the upper torso, the woman is effectively adopting the yogic pose known as the "upward-facing dog". Although it doesn't sound very flattering, this pose stretches the chest and abdominals, strengthens the spine, and improves posture. Remember, ladies, if it's great for your posture, it's great for your breasts.

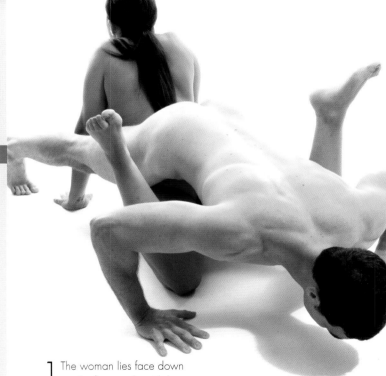

1 The woman lies face down on the floor and—with her hands placed shoulder-width apart—extends her arms to raise her torso. The man adopts a similar push-up position facing in the opposite direct to his partner with his legs open as he enters her from behind.

2 The woman then flexes her thighs to raise her lower legs so that the man can place his hands further apart (the wide positioning of the hands increases the use of the chest muscles as opposed to the arm muscles).

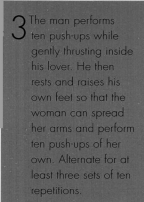

3 The man performs ten push-ups while gently thrusting inside his lover. He then rests and raises his own feet so that the woman can spread her arms and perform ten push-ups of her own. Alternate for at least three sets of ten repetitions.

HOT TIP

The extreme angle of entry makes vaginal penetration tricky, to say the least, and for fans of anal sex this sexercise is easier to perform with anal penetration.

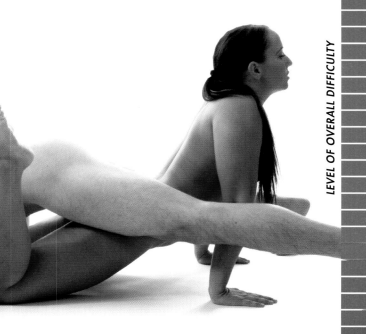

HARD

LEVEL OF OVERALL DIFFICULTY

EASY

PLANKS FOR THE MAMMARIES

Look familiar? This sexercise basically combines push-ups for her with triceps dips for him. Once again, the guy gets to enjoy a great view of his partner's sexy ass as she works out but, unfortunately for him, he can only look and lust as his hands remain planted firmly on the ground when they really want to be wandering over her rump. This sexercise provides a really vigorous workout for the woman's pectorals, but it's also a great overall fitness routine.

MAJOR TARGETS

Pectorals	Pectorals
Triceps	Triceps
Deltoids	Deltoids

HOT TIP

For a great triceps workout—and to help his partner keep her body as straight as possible while she performs her push-ups—the man should lower his torso as she lowers hers, until he feels a gentle stretch in his shoulders. As she pushes up once more, he pushes his own body up until his arms are once again straight.

1 The man adopts an upward-facing plank position with his arms and legs fully extended. His partner mounts him facing in the opposite direction with her arms and legs extended in the standard push-up position.

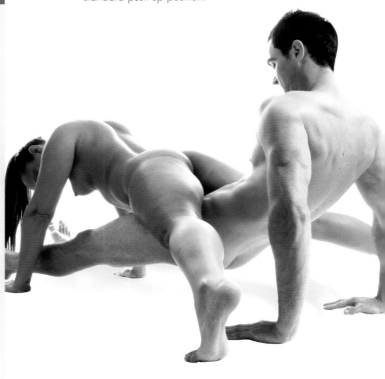

2 The woman then performs a set of eight to ten push-ups, keeping her body as straight as possible.

HOT TIP

If the female partner finds this routine too difficult to maintain, she can move into a squatting position to allow him to continue his sexercise while she still gets to work her legs. If he is the one struggling, he can simply place his butt on the floor and, quite literally, sit it out while she finishes up her routine.

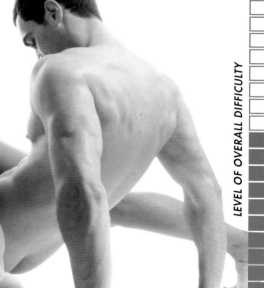

LEVEL OF OVERALL DIFFICULTY

HARD

EASY

GATOR LAID

While the woman focuses on her pectoralis-minor muscles with subtle movements of her shoulders, the man is effectively adopting the yogic upward-facing dog—stretching his pectoralis-major muscles and working on a host of other muscle groups in his upper leg, butt, and torso, including the spinal-erector muscles that are crucial to good posture. He'll also have to exercise his self-control, this is a relatively easy sexercise but one that is highly stimulating for him particularly.

MAJOR TARGETS

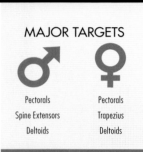

♂ | ♀

Pectorals	Pectorals
Spine Extensors	Trapezius
Deltoids	Deltoids

HOT TIP

This is a great position to slow things down during a workout. The man is in the perfect position to plant kisses on her highly sexually sensitive neck, shoulders, and earlobes.

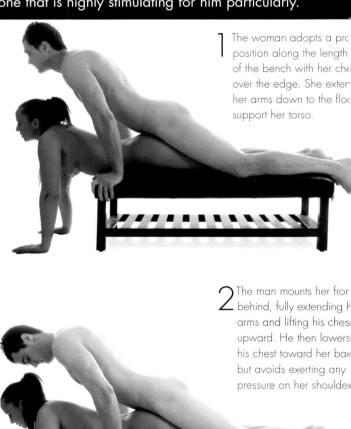

1 The woman adopts a pro position along the length of the bench with her che over the edge. She exter her arms down to the floo support her torso.

2 The man mounts her fror behind, fully extending h arms and lifting his ches upward. He then lowers his chest toward her ba but avoids exerting any pressure on her shoulde

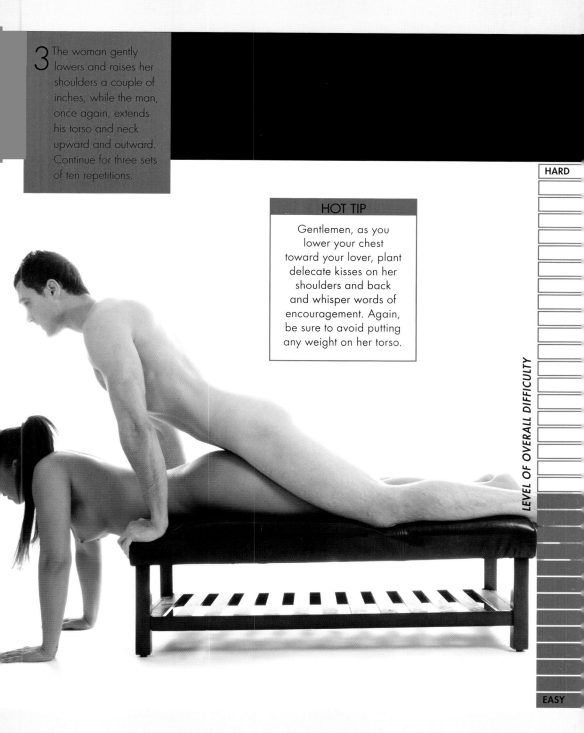

3 The woman gently lowers and raises her shoulders a couple of inches, while the man, once again, extends his torso and neck upward and outward. Continue for three sets of ten repetitions.

HOT TIP

Gentlemen, as you lower your chest toward your lover, plant delicate kisses on her shoulders and back and whisper words of encouragement. Again, be sure to avoid putting any weight on her torso.

LEVEL OF OVERALL DIFFICULTY

HARD

EASY

HARD CORE

This is a relatively easy session and, while you will certainly feel the burn in your core abdominal muscles, the woman will be so distracted by what he is doing with his tongue that she won't want to stop. So while she stretches forward and backward in increasing ecstasy for ten minutes or longer, he performs his part of the bargain for, what... a couple of hundred laps maybe?

MAJOR TARGETS

Deltoids	Abdominals
Abdominals	Deltoids
Pectorals	Pectorals

HOT TIP

If either partner becomes tired then feel free to rest in the fully prone positions and focus on the oral fun for a while. That way he can release his hands for a couple of minutes to help explore her most intimate areas. You'll quickly find yourselves relaxed and raring to go for rounds two and three.

1 The woman gets on all fours while resting on her forearms with her hands clasped in front of her.

2 The man adopts a similar position directly behind her with his hands placed on either side of her lower thighs and administers oral pleasure.

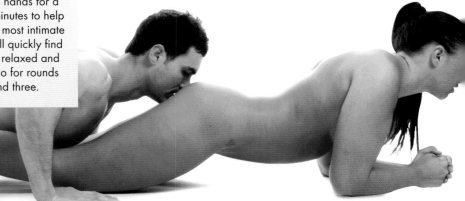

3 She stretches forward and down and he follows her, all the while maintaining contact orally. She then stretches back up into the original position and the process is repeated. Repeat the sexercise for ten to fifteen minutes in two or three five-minute sessions.

HOT TIP

Some men will love to exchange roles in this position. Although she won't be able to give him full-on oral sex, she will be able to lightly flick her tongue over his testicles—a compromise that is certainly not to be sniffed at.

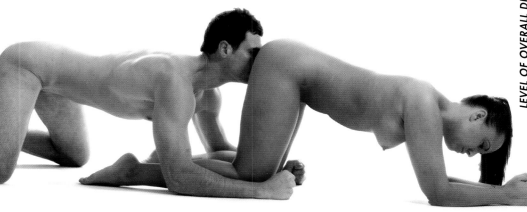

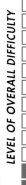

PARK AND RIDE

This is a hot favorite among male sexercise aficionados as it provides satisfying sexual stimulation and a great view of her ass. It's also an excellent full-body workout for him as he uses muscles from his neck all the way down to his toes. On that note, for all you female foot-fetishists out there, this the perfect opportunity to indulge in a bit of toe-sucking and general foot worship.

MAJOR TARGETS

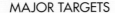

Pectorals	Pectorals
Abdominals	Triceps
Triceps	Deltoids

HOT TIP

While the man is thrusting up from behind, the woman can coax him by reaching behind from the kneeling position to cup and fondle his testicles with light touches and the occasional gentle squeeze.

1 The man sits on the floor or bed while the woman kneels in front of him facing in the same direction and mounts his penis.

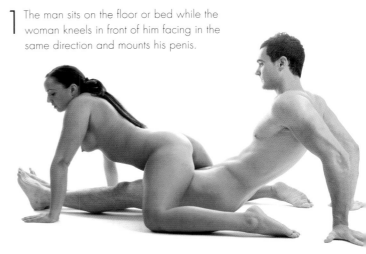

2 As the woman leans forward on all fours, the man raises his hips off the floor to stay inside her, taking his weight on his arms and fully opening his chest.

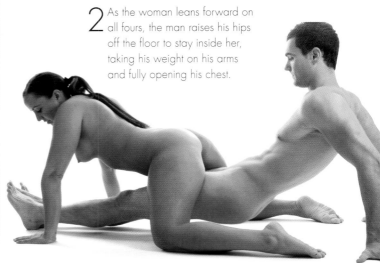

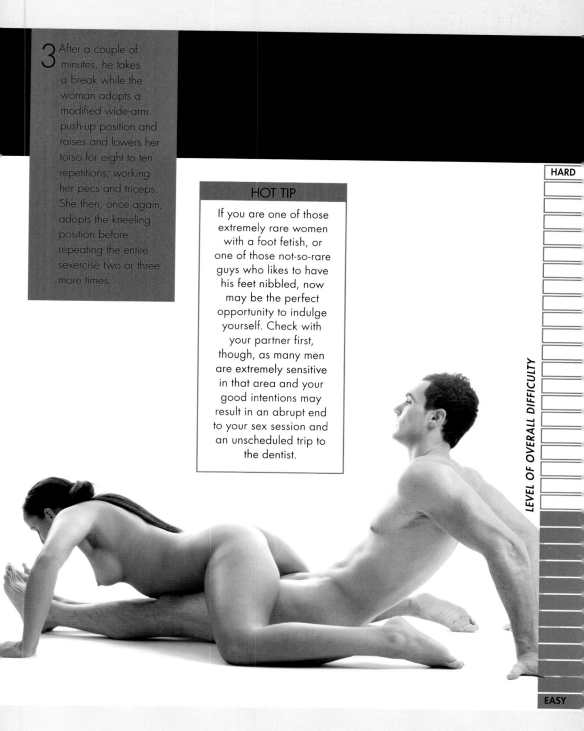

3 After a couple of minutes, he takes a break while the woman adopts a modified wide-arm push-up position and raises and lowers her torso for eight to ten repetitions, working her pecs and triceps. She then, once again, adopts the kneeling position before repeating the entire sexercise two or three more times.

HOT TIP

If you are one of those extremely rare women with a foot fetish, or one of those not-so-rare guys who likes to have his feet nibbled, now may be the perfect opportunity to indulge yourself. Check with your partner first, though, as many men are extremely sensitive in that area and your good intentions may result in an abrupt end to your sex session and an unscheduled trip to the dentist.

HARD

LEVEL OF OVERALL DIFFICULTY

EASY

THE PEARL DIVER

Perhaps not surprisingly, this position is a hot favorite among female aficionados of sexercise: Initially, she gets to work those inner-thigh muscles by spreading her legs outward then drawing them back toward her partners face; then, by raising herself into the bridge position, she works her legs, butt, back, shoulders, arms, and chest—the full monty. All this while her lover devotes his full attention to her labia and clitoris.

MAJOR TARGETS

Triceps	Quadriceps
Pectorals	Glutes
Hamstrings	Pectorals

HOT TIP

For him, too, this is a full-body workout with all the benefits of the push-up-type exercises, while giving his lover great oral sex.

1 The woman positions herself on the floor in a supine position with her arms by her side. She brings her feet back halfway toward her butt.

2 From a kneeling position, with a knee placed either side of her head, he leans forward and places a hand on each side of her hips. The man then pushes up into a modified plank position with his arms bent and butt raised and pleasures her orally.

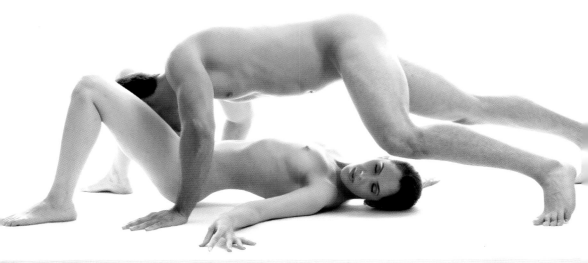

3 Using her shoulders and feet as levers, the woman then raises her hips to adopt a bridge position. As she lifts her hips, the man extends his arms to continue administering oral sex. Aim to complete at least three sets of ten bridge raises.

HOT TIP

Sexercise aficionados are a sharing, caring community; the woman can give a little back while relaxing between sets. After all, she's only a few inches away from the famous and fabulous 69 sex position.

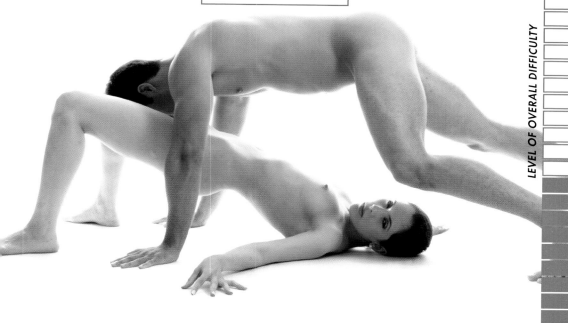

LEVEL OF OVERALL DIFFICULTY

HARD

EASY

THREE BALLS AND A BAT

Of all the incentives ever provided for a guy to do push-ups this has got them all beat hands down. Each time he lowers himself toward the floor he gets to feel his lover's lips close around the head of his penis—he'll be breaking his own personal best every week. For her, it's admittedly not so much of a workout as a well-earned rest and a chance to reward her lover for his pearl-diving exploits (see p50.).

MAJOR TARGETS

Pectorals	Platysma
Triceps	Masseter
Abdominals	Glossus

HOT TIP

For the woman, this is a great opportunity to work those oft-neglected muscles in the neck, jaw, and, yes, the tongue. By basically pulling funny faces and extending your tongue fully (don't worry he isn't looking—he has his mind on other things) you are working the platysma, which is a thin, flat muscles that covers the front of the neck and which helps you keep a firm, sleek throat, as opposed to a sagging, wrinkly one, plus a host of other muscles in the jaw and tongue.

1 The woman positions herself on the floor in a supine position with her arms by her side. She brings her feet back halfway toward her butt.

2 The man adopts a push-up position—here, using a small stability ball to really focus the work on the pecs and triceps.

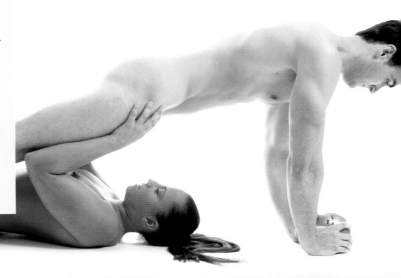

3 As the man keeps his body straight and lowers his chest toward the floor, the woman slowly curls her shoulders, neck, and head off the floor while tensing her abdominal muscles. Continue for at least three sets of ten push-ups.

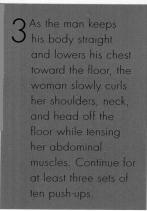

HOT TIP

For women who want to keep working out, this is a great opportunity to work the lower abdominals by putting her legs together and raising her knees toward her partner's butt. She then lowers her knees and straightens her legs while keeping her heels a couple of inches off the floor. If she repeats this action a dozen or so times without touching the ground she will really start to feel the burn in her abdominals.

HARD

LEVEL OF OVERALL DIFFICULTY

EASY

CHEST WORKOUT 1

This workout combines four sexercises that will help him develop strong, firm pectoral muscles that will look great in a t-shirt, and help her keep her breasts high and perky.

THE DOUBLE UP (pages 40–41)

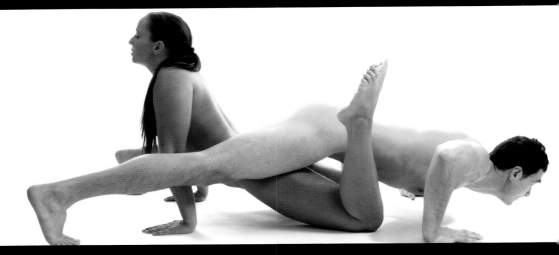

PLANKS FOR THE MAMMARIES (pages 42–43)

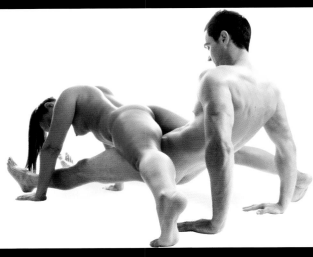

DURATION
Perform each position for
2 minutes minimum, increasing 30
seconds per additional workout

SCHEDULE
Once every other week

PARK AND RIDE (pages 48–49)

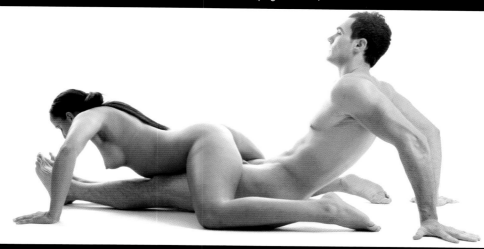

GATOR LAID (pages 44–45)

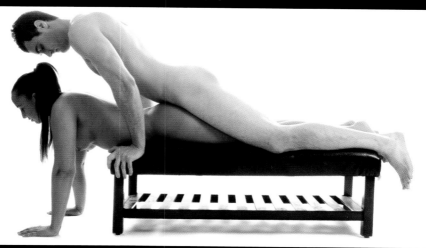

CHEST WORKOUT 2

This workout combines four sexercises that focus on the chest. As well as working those pectorals, this offers the opportunity for some fabulous oral sex.

THREE BALLS AND A BAT (pages 52–53)

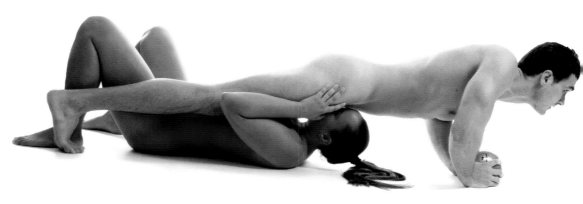

HARD CORE (pages 46–47)

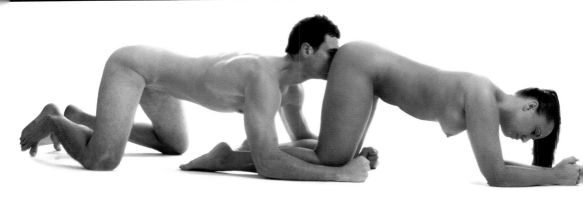

THE PEARL DIVER (pages 50–51)

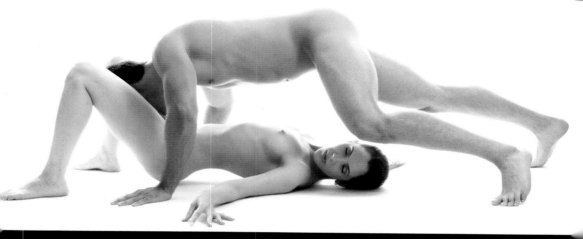

DO THE LOTION MOTION (pages 134–35)

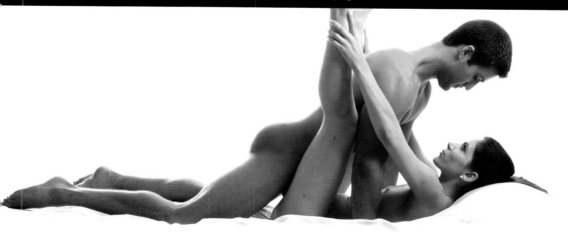

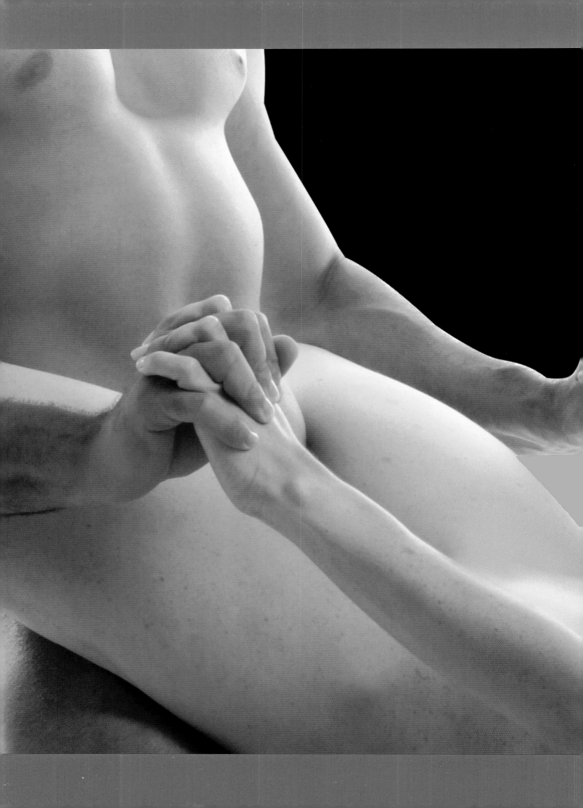

ALLURING ABS

Great Abs are the core of great physical fitness and we love them because they help to keep the stomach lean and flat. In a superfit body they create the classic "six-pack" that all men long for and all women lust after. But the "core muscles" aren't just the abs; they are a whole bunch of muscles that stabilize the spine, hips, and shoulder-girdle to create a solid support base for the entire body. For great sex, make no mistake, the core muscles are the most important group of all, making us flexible, strong, ready for action, and—perhaps most importantly—reducing the strain on the spine in more extreme positions. Having said that, a lot of core exercises are about small, subtle movements zoning in on key muscles, so this chapter contains some relatively low-key sexercises that offer great opportunities for the softer side of sex: erotic massage and the kissing and canoodling that makes good sex glorious.

THE AB ARCH

Once again, the challenge here is to keep the penis inserted, so be aware that only very small movements are required to target the abs and related core muscles. For the woman, this bridge position is also great for the glutes and thighs. For the man, this kneeling position really gets to work on the hip-flexors. By stretching his torso upward and back, and extending his neck, he can also target the glutes and trapezius.

MAJOR TARGETS

♂	♀
Abdominals	Abdominals
Hip Flexors	Glutes
Hamstrings	Quadriceps

HOT TIP

By placing his hands behind his back between his partner's feet and extending his torso further, the guy can work his lower back and spinal extensors. By placing a single hand behind his back, he can twist his body to work his obliques. He should swap arms every minute or so to work the obliques on the opposite side of his torso.

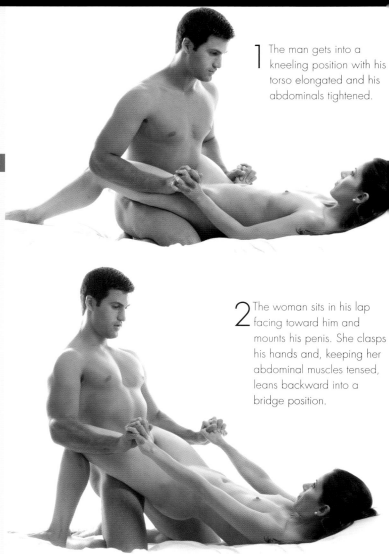

1 The man gets into a kneeling position with his torso elongated and his abdominals tightened.

2 The woman sits in his lap facing toward him and mounts his penis. She clasps his hands and, keeping her abdominal muscles tensed, leans backward into a bridge position.

3 The man makes small thrusting motions with his hips while the woman responds by lifting her pelvis in similarly subtle movements. Continue for at least ten minutes.

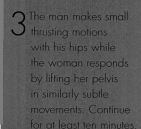

HOT TIP

This is another position where the guy is offered a wonderful view of his lover's breasts. Let go of one of his hands and fondle your breasts to raise the temperature a little further. Then guide his other hand toward an anatomical area of your choice...decisions, decisions.

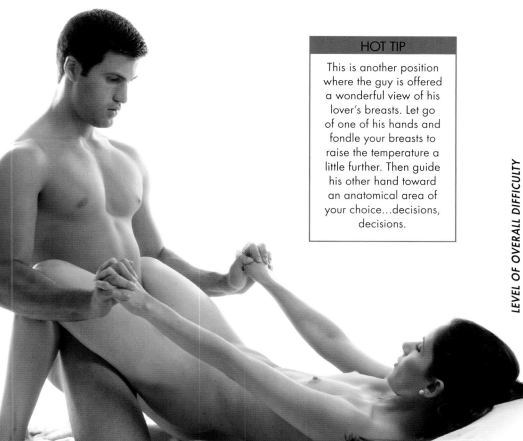

LEVEL OF OVERALL DIFFICULTY

HARD

EASY

THE TWISTED SISTER

This is an especially good workout for the woman's abs and obliques as she twists toward her partner to allow him to enter her; but it is also a good overall workout for her shoulders, back, and arms. He also works his abs as he lifts her gently up and down, plus he gets all the benefits of the squat, which is a great workout for the legs and glutes. It is important to repeat the sexercise from the opposite side so that both sets of oblique muscles are worked evenly.

MAJOR TARGETS

♂

| Abdominals |
| Glutes |
| Hamstrings |

♀

| Obliques |
| Abdominals |
| Trapezius |

HOT TIP

The man can adapt this position to work his arms and upper back by slowly "shrugging" his shoulder up and down to raise and lower his partner, especially targeting his deltoids, triceps, and trapezius.

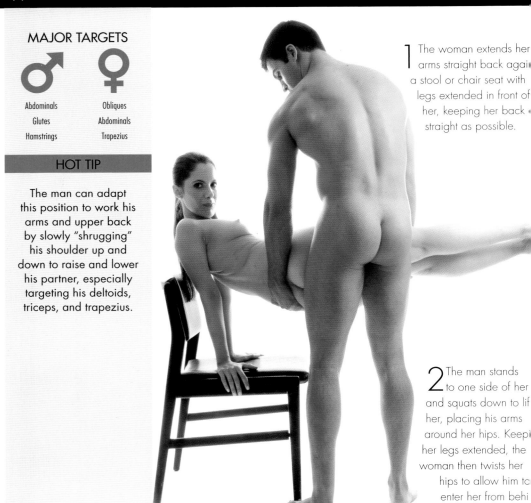

1 The woman extends her arms straight back agai a stool or chair seat with legs extended in front of her, keeping her back straight as possible.

2 The man stands to one side of her and squats down to lif her, placing his arms around her hips. Keepi her legs extended, the woman then twists her hips to allow him to enter her from behi

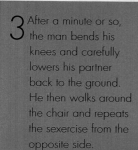

3 After a minute or so, the man bends his knees and carefully lowers his partner back to the ground. He then walks around the chair and repeats the sexercise from the opposite side.

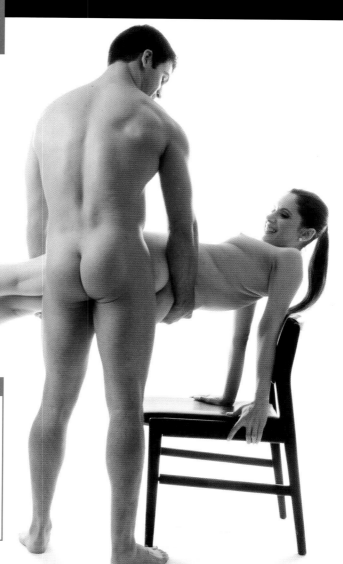

HOT TIP

For the man who prefers rear-entry sex, this is and exciting and novel approach to backdoor sex that allows the man to view his lover's fantastic breasts without resorting to the strategic placement of mirrors.

LEVEL OF OVERALL DIFFICULTY

HARD

EASY

YUMMY TUMMIES

Here's a position where the guy really gets to enjoy the fruits of her labors as he relishes the view and reaches forward to run his hands over that beautifully toned belly and waspish waist. He doesn't get to relax too much, however, as the action of stretching forward should be performed as a "crunch," working his abdominal muscles. By arching back from a kneeling position, the woman is getting a more vigorous workout of her abdominals and pectorals.

MAJOR TARGETS

Abdominals	Abdominals
Trapezius	Hip Flexors
Deltoids	Trapezius

HOT TIP

This woman-on-top position is a great opportunity for her to titillate and tease her partner as she tweaks and fondles her breasts, while keeping them tantalizingly out of reach. If she's feeling generous, she can put him out of his misery by raising her body and leaning forward to allow him to fondle her breasts and suck her nipples before, once again, leaning back and continuing the sexercise.

1 The man lies back on the bed in a fully extended supine posture and the woman mounts him in a kneeling position and reclines against his legs.

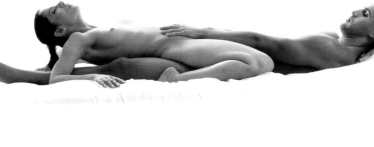

2 She then slowly raises her torso toward her lover by supporting her weight on both hands, feeling the intense stretch in her abdominal muscles.

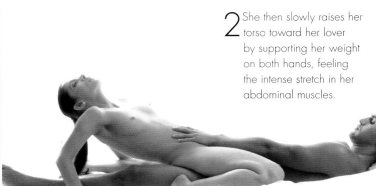

3 The woman fully extends her arms and stretches her neck back, while the man performs continuous crunches. She raises and lowers her arms for at least fifteen repetitions before reclining fully against his legs. She should aim to complete three sets of fifteen repetitions.

HOT TIP

By leaning fully back against his legs she is really working those abs, as well as her quadriceps and a host of other muscles. She is also giving him, quite literally, an open invitation to stroke her clitoris.

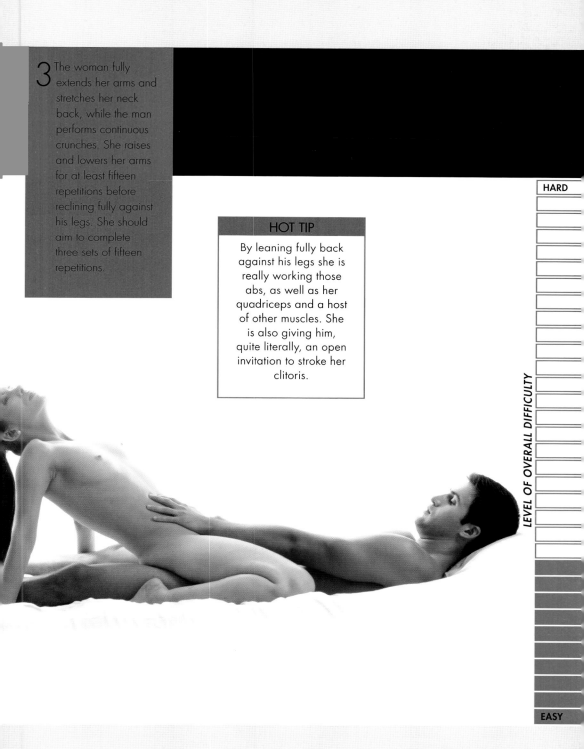

LEVEL OF OVERALL DIFFICULTY

HARD

EASY

THE DOUBLE CRUNCH

This sexercise will look very familiar to fit folk who will immediately recognize the "crunch" and will know just how effective it is for sculpting a sensational six-pack. And he doesn't need a spotter to encourage him to do "just one more"—he has all the encouragement he needs as each time he sits up he's rewarded with the view of his lover's gorgeous butt rising and falling on his penis. Meanwhile, the woman performs a more concentrated crunch of her own.

MAJOR TARGETS

Abdominals	Abdominals
Trapezius	Spine Extensors
Deltoids	Hip Flexors

HOT TIP

For the guy particularly, there is the opportunity for endless variations on this exercise. He can, for example, change to twisting crunches (twisting his torso to one side and then the other as he sits up) to work his obliques. Or, he can work a completely different muscle group by using dumbbells to perform "flies"—holding a weight in each hand with arms extended directly above the chest, then lowering the arms to each side until the stretch is felt in the chest before returning to the starting position.

1 The man sits down on the end of an exercise bench with his feet flat on the floor and leans back into a supine position. The woman mounts him in a seated position facing away from her partner.

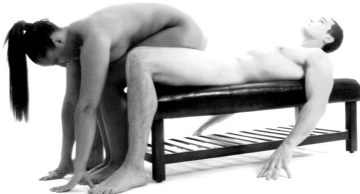

2 The woman then stretches her hands down toward the ground and places her hands behind her ankles gently pulling her body downward while tightening her abdominal muscles.

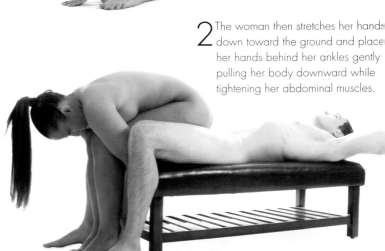

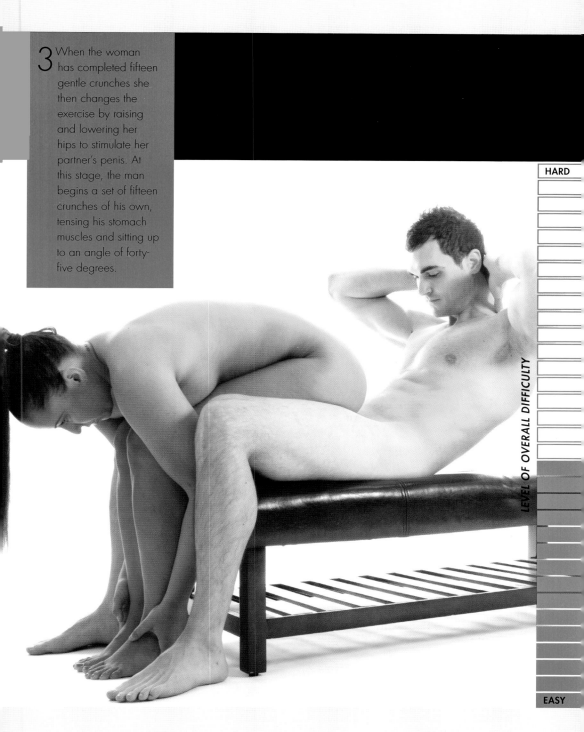

3 When the woman has completed fifteen gentle crunches she then changes the exercise by raising and lowering her hips to stimulate her partner's penis. At this stage, the man begins a set of fifteen crunches of his own, tensing his stomach muscles and sitting up to an angle of forty-five degrees.

HARD

LEVEL OF OVERALL DIFFICULTY

EASY

MIRROR, MIRROR

A fabulous and fun workout for the core muscles, you can introduce an element of healthy competition as one partner takes a turn to set the pace while the other aims to mirror every move. Being on top, the woman will feel the stretch more intensely as she leans back after completing each set of crunches. Make sure that the actual crunch movements are relatively small (don't recline backward fully each time) so that you really target those abdominal muscles.

MAJOR TARGETS

Abdominals	Abdominals
Trapezius	Spine Extensors
Deltoids	Hip Flexors

HOT TIP

Unless your partner happens to be hung like a horse, it is very difficult for him to keep his penis inserted when reclining back at the end of each set. So, simply sit up and climb back on board before restarting each set. It's worth the effort; make a habit of this great sexercise and you will soon have the fairest abs of all.

1 The man sits down with a leg on either side of an exercise bench and his lover mounts him facing in the opposite direction.

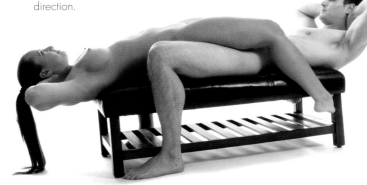

2 Both partners then lie back and place their hands up behind their heads. They then flex and twist the waist to raise the upper torso performing twisting crunches to opposite sides.

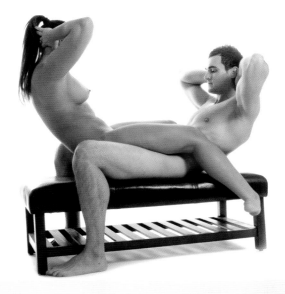

3 Complete at least ten crunches to each side—with only small movements of the torso—before reclining back into the starting position. Aim to complete at least three sets of ten repetitions.

HOT TIP

As a face-to-face sexercise, don't resist the urge to make out at the end of each set and give a little exercise to those oft-neglected but all-important jaw and tongue muscles.

HARD

LEVEL OF OVERALL DIFFICULTY

EASY

FANCY FOOTWORK

OK, this sexercise clearly demonstrates that you don't have to adopt extreme positions to give your abdominals a good workout. This modified missionary position is as tame and tender as lovemaking gets and yet—by simply arching her pelvis up to meet him—she can be working her hip flexors and abdominals while focusing full attention on her lover. By thrusting forward from the prone position, the guy works his abdominals and hip flexors too.

MAJOR TARGETS

Abdominals	Abdominals
Hip Flexors	Hip Flexors
Deltoids	Hamstrings

HOT TIP

The woman can make this a more energetic workout by getting creative with her legs. She has all that fancy footwork to think about as she caresses his muscular calves with the soles of her feet but she is also free to raise her legs in the air or clasp her partner around the waist to give her own thighs and glutes a real burn.

1 The woman lies in a supine position and man adopts a prone position on top. She wraps her thighs around his and places her feet on his lower legs. Using her feet and shoulders as levers, she arches her back and he enters her.

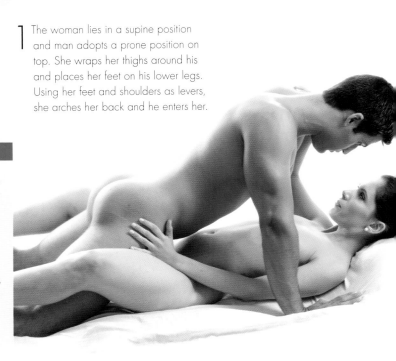

2 The woman holds the arch for at least two minutes then she relaxes back onto the bed. The man, in turn, tightens his abdominals and arches forward to continue making love. Meanwhile, the woman focuses on her thigh muscles by clasping him with her thighs and running her feet along his calves.

3 After another couple of minutes, the woman arches her back once more and restarts the cycle. Continue for at least ten minutes.

HOT TIP

Gentlemen, while she is arching her hips toward you, you can work you arms and chest by lowering your torso towards hers. While you're at it, you can take her mind off the exercise aspect by whispering "sweet nothings"—or talking dirty— whatever works for you guys.

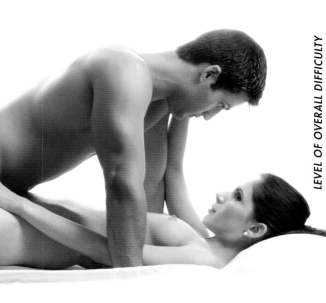

HARD

LEVEL OF OVERALL DIFFICULTY

EASY

BENT BUDS

The extreme angle of entry makes this sexercise difficult to complete successfully without the penis continually slipping out. The trick is to move very slowly, keeping the abdominal muscles contracted and moving in perfect synchronization. The man might find it easier to enter her initially at the arched stage of this sexercise, before lowering down into the prone position. When this sexercise works, the sexual pleasure is very intense as both partners focus so directly on the genital area.

MAJOR TARGETS

♂	♀
Abdominals	Abdominals
Hip Flexors	Hip Flexors
Deltoids	Hamstrings

HOT TIP

The woman can help by contracting her pelvic-floor muscles to grip the head of his penis as he rises up into the arched posture.

1 The woman lies face down with her forearms on the floor, elbows bent, and palms flat. The man adopts a similar position facing in the opposite direction and enters her.

2 Very slowly and carefully, bracing himself on his forearms and toes, the man raises his body into a modified plank position, while the woman raises her hips so that his penis remains inside her.

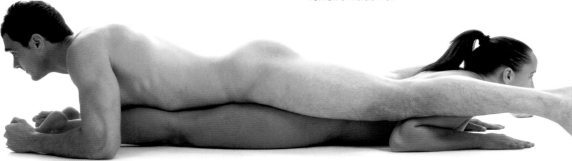

3 With equal care, the partners lower themselves back into the original position, all the while focusing on keeping the abdominal muscles tight. Repeat three or four times.

HOT TIP

For those who enjoy sex via the "back door," anal penetration can be easier than vaginal penetration in this workout.

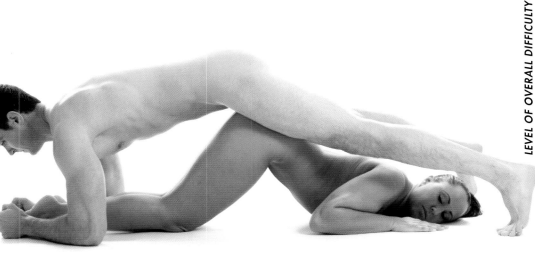

LEVEL OF OVERALL DIFFICULTY

HARD

EASY

CORE BLASTER

As its name suggests, this sexercise is a great overall workout for the core-muscle group, especially for the woman in this instance. As she arches her body upward, she is activating her entire core to maintain stability. As she lowers her torso, she should really feel the stretch in her inner thighs and upper back. For him, this is also a great ab workout, but he's also working his glutes and upper thighs, keeping that butt looking great.

MAJOR TARGETS

Abdominals	Abdominals
Glutes	Spine Extensors
Quadriceps	Obliques

HOT TIP

By raising her thigh, the woman can vary the angle of entry to maximize her sexual pleasure and enjoy really deep penetration in this position.

1 The woman lies face up on the floor with her feet resting on a chair or the end of a bed. The man then stands over her with his feet placed on either side of her hips.

2 Using her hands and feet as levers, the woman pushes herself up into an inverted-plank position. She then raises her left leg onto his shoulder. The man supports her hips and enters her.

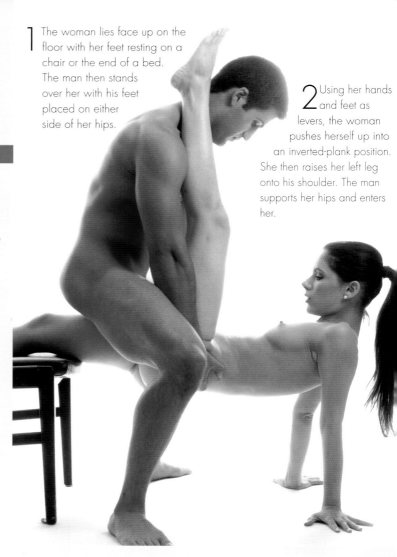

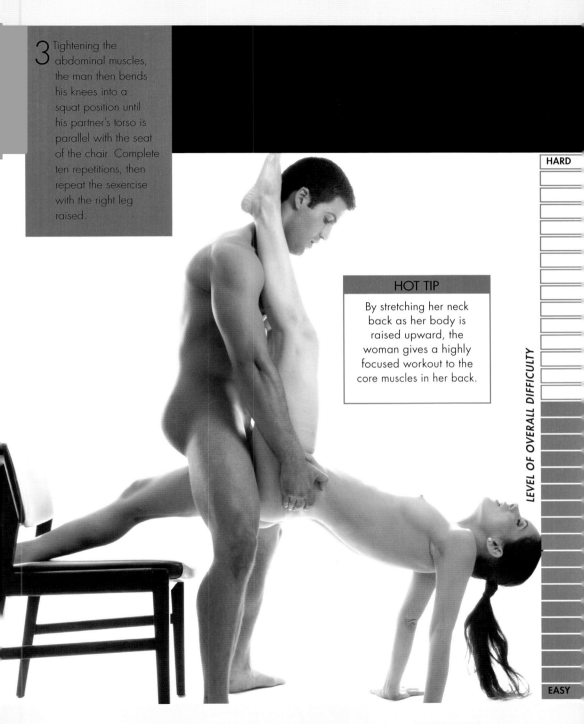

3 Tightening the abdominal muscles, the man then bends his knees into a squat position until his partner's torso is parallel with the seat of the chair. Complete ten repetitions, then repeat the sexercise with the right leg raised.

HOT TIP

By stretching her neck back as her body is raised upward, the woman gives a highly focused workout to the core muscles in her back.

LEVEL OF OVERALL DIFFICULTY

HARD

EASY

ABS WORKOUT 1

This workout combines four relatively gentle sexercises that you can enjoy without any props or acrobatics, while still whittling away at that waistline by working your abdominal muscles.

FANCY FOOTWORK (pages 70–71)

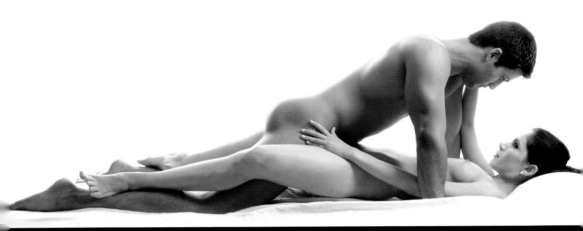

THE AB ARCH (pages 60–61)

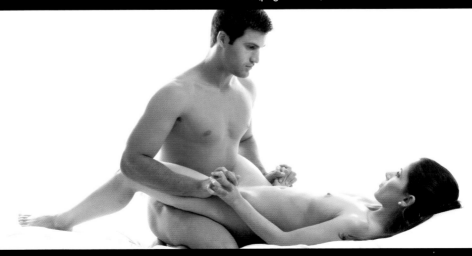

YUMMY TUMMIES (pages 64–65)

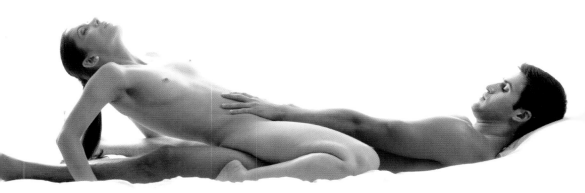

THE SQUAT THRUST (pages 96–97)

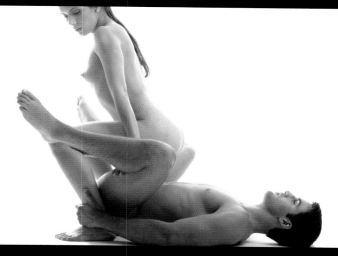

ABS WORKOUT 2

This more vigorous workout combines four fab sexercises that focus intensely on the entire core. You will need a chair or exercise bench to complete the workout.

CORE BLASTER
(pages 74–75)

THE TWISTED SISTER
(pages 62–63)

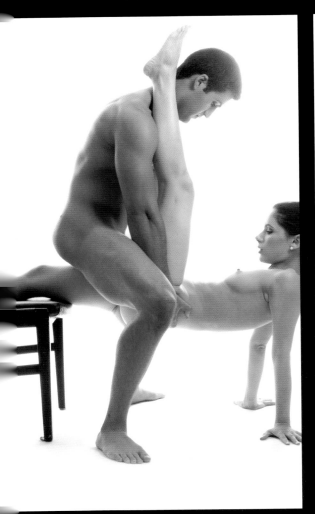

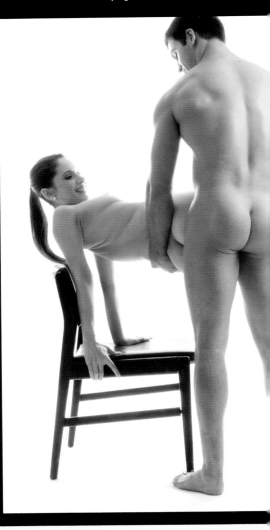

DURATION
Perform each position for
2 minutes minimum, increasing 30
seconds per additional workout

SCHEDULE
Once every other week

MIRROR, MIRROR (pages 68–69)

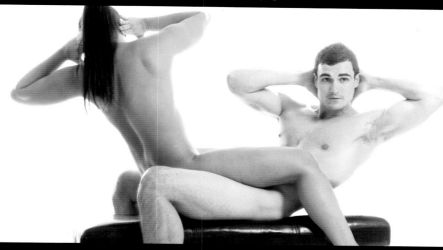

THE DOUBLE CRUNCH (pages 66–67)

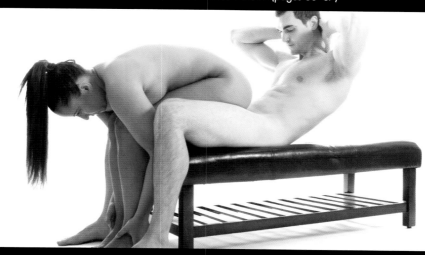

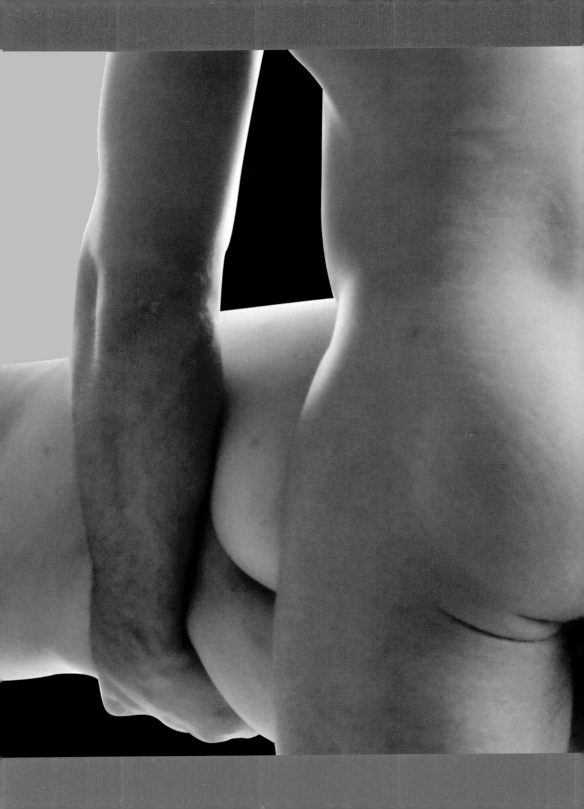

BEAUTIFUL BUTTS

f a woman's breasts are magnets for a guy's eyes when face to face with a woman, from a rear view it is a woman's butt that exerts the main gravitational pull. Women are divided on the issue as far as ogling guys from behind is concerned—a guy's broad shoulders and a classically V-shaped back are often awarded higher pulling points than his ass. But, guys, even if you're as broad as a barn in the shoulder region, it's no good if your ass is similarly proportioned. So, either way, men need to work out on the core muscles and glutes to look great from behind. When we're talking sex, the butt's importance is a no-brainer. All that bumping and grinding requires a guy to possess powerful glutes. For a woman, it's not so much power she's looking for as shapeliness and firmness—keeping her butt cheeks high, toned, and firm. All of the sexercises in this chapter will assist her in that noble endeavor.

GLUTE AWAKENING

In this compact position it is really easy for him to focus on his glutes, and he'll soon feel the burn that tells him they're getting a great workout. He's also getting an excellent workout on his hamstrings, shoulders, and triceps. The woman gets her workout by resisting the pressure of his hips, while concentrating on clenching her butt cheeks and holding on to the chair seat to steady herself as he thrusts.

MAJOR TARGETS

Glutes	Abdominals
Hip Flexors	Glutes
Hamstrings	Quadriceps

HOT TIP

For her, it may not be so easy to connect mind to muscle on this one. My advice is, the first couple of times you try this sexercise, imagine that you're holding a dollar coin between your butt cheeks and you're trying not to let it fall (not the sexiest image, I know, but it gets you targeting the right muscles).

1 The man sits on a sturdy chair and, bracing his arms against the back of the seat, raises his heels up onto the edge of the seat.

2 His partner stands with he back toward him and, wit her hands placed upon hi knees, lowers herself onto his penis.

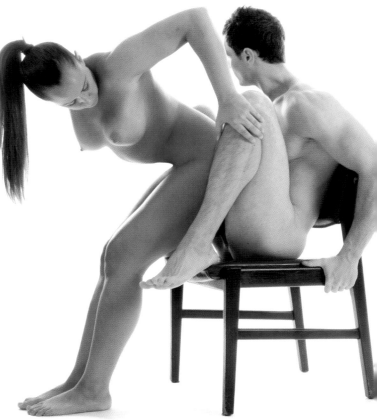

3 As he raises his butt and thrusts, she tightens and releases her glutes. Aim to continue for at least ten minutes.

HOT TIP

If the woman is a fan of anal sex, you can bring a dildo into play to liven up proceedings.

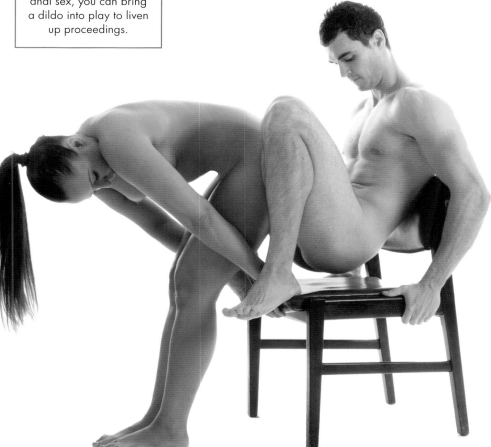

LEVEL OF OVERALL DIFFICULTY

HARD

EASY

LIMBO LUST

Limbo lust provides a wonderful workout for the woman's glutes, especially as she does most of the work in terms of bump and grind despite his being on top. This sexercise actually works her entire core but it is the burn in her chest and shoulders that will bring the first passage of play to a close. He gets to work his glutes when he lowers her to the ground and takes over the pump action but he, too, will feel the burn in his chest, shoulders, and arms.

MAJOR TARGETS

Deltoids	Glutes
Core Muscles	Pectorals
Glutes	Deltoids

HOT TIP

You may find it easier to begin this sexercise from a seated position. The guy sits in a chair and the woman sits in his lap facing toward him. He then gets up and kneels on the floor while she clings on to him with her core and butt muscles tightened.

1 The woman lies on the floor or bed in a supine position with her legs parted and knees bent. The man kneels between her thighs and leans forward into a kneeling push-up position.

2 The man bends his arms and presses his chest against her breasts. She then clasps her arms around his upper body and, placing her feet on either side of his thighs, raises her hips to allow him to enter her. He performs five push-ups.

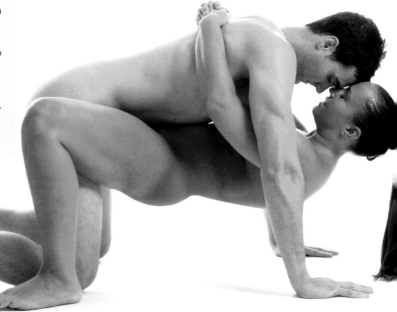

3 The woman then contracts her glutes and thrusts her hips. After a minute or so, the man lowers his chest toward the floor and thrusts for one minute before raising his chest once more to restart the cycle. Repeat the cycle at least two or three times.

HOT TIP

If the woman is small compared to her guy she can give him the maximum upper-body workout by shifting into full bush-baby mode, wrapping her thighs around his lower back so that she is completely suspended—a great workout for her thighs.

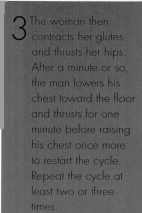

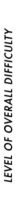

HARD

LEVEL OF OVERALL DIFFICULTY

EASY

BUMPING RUMPS

This time around, it's the guy who gets the better butt workout while the woman lies back and focuses on working her pelvic-floor muscles to create really explosive sensations in her lover's penis—contorted as it is in this unusual position. She should also tighten her glutes and abs to feel—and supply—a real squeeze in her nether regions. He, meanwhile, gets to play hippity hoppity while watching the big game on cable TV.

MAJOR TARGETS

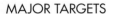

Glutes	Glutes
Hamstrings	Pelvic Floor
Quadriceps	Quadriceps

HOT TIP

The woman may find this easier, and make it easier for him, if she clasps her own thighs beneath her knees and pulls her legs toward her chest.

1 The woman lies on the floor in a supine position with her legs raised and parted, and her knees bent. The man squats between her thighs and enters her.

2 As the woman focuses on tightening her glutes and pelvic-floor muscles, the man raises and lowers his hips in a gentle bouncing action. Continue for at least five minutes.

HOT TIP

My alternative title for this is the Isaac Murphy, named after the great American jockey. As a very constricting and impersonal position it appeals to women who enjoy bondage play so you might want to spice things up by getting your whip out before heading for the home straight—always assuming that your little pony approves, of course. Bear in mind, though, that this can work two ways, so she might prefer to be the one wielding the whip.

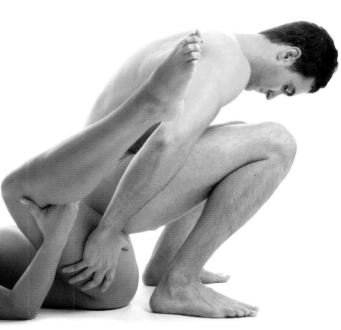

HARD

LEVEL OF OVERALL DIFFICULTY

EASY

MOUNT PLEASANT

The bridge pose is a classic yogic posture that provides an excellent full-body workout but, given the amount of muscle actions that need to be balanced to maintain this pose correctly, a high degree of coordination is required. If, as the guy, you're fortunate enough to have a partner who is proficient at yoga then this is very pleasant sexercise indeed, allowing deep penetration that can bring you to the summit of sexual pleasure—and you get to plant your flagpole before even leaving base camp.

MAJOR TARGETS

♂

| Glutes |
| Hip Flexors |
| Abdominals |

♀

| Glutes |
| Hamstrings |
| Quadriceps |

HOT TIP

As the woman relaxes down onto her partner's thighs, he can apply manual stimulation to her clitoris to heighten her sexual arousal.

1 The woman lies on the floor in a supine position with her legs bent and arms outstretched. Using her shoulders and feet as levers, she raises herself into a bridge positic

2 The man kneels between her thighs and, placing his hands on either side of her hips, enters her and makes long, even, thrusting strokes while focusing on tightening his glutes.

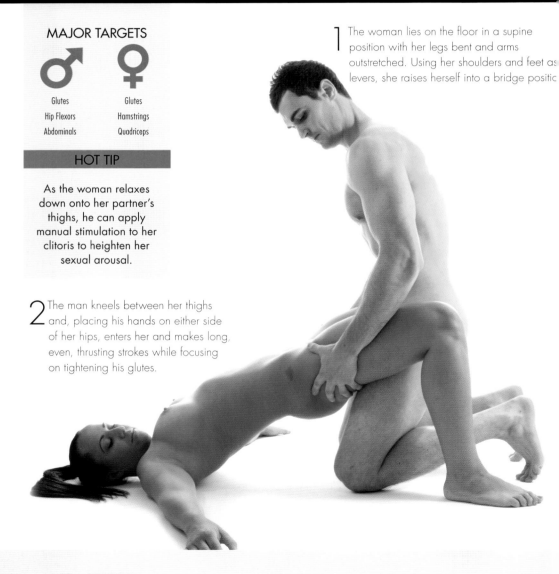

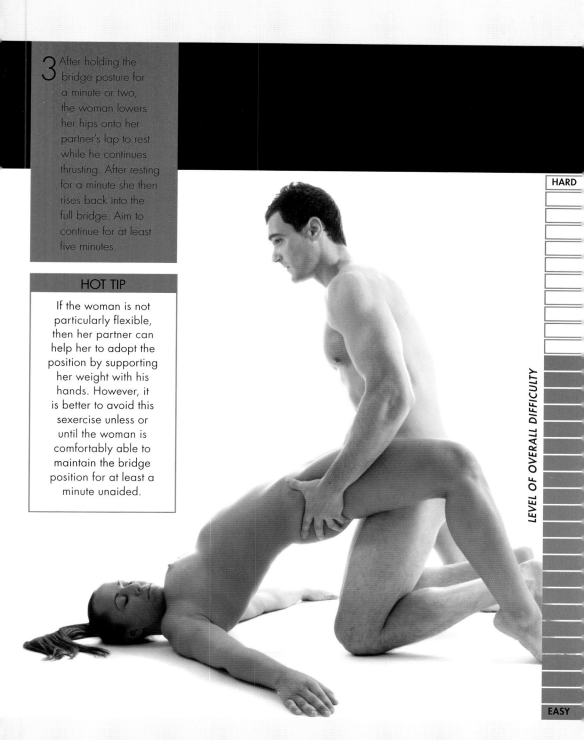

3 After holding the bridge posture for a minute or two, the woman lowers her hips onto her partner's lap to rest while he continues thrusting. After resting for a minute she then rises back into the full bridge. Aim to continue for at least five minutes.

HOT TIP

If the woman is not particularly flexible, then her partner can help her to adopt the position by supporting her weight with his hands. However, it is better to avoid this sexercise unless or until the woman is comfortably able to maintain the bridge position for at least a minute unaided.

LEVEL OF OVERALL DIFFICULTY

HARD

EASY

SUMMER OF LOVE

By all accounts '69 was a vintage year for love and, as we all know, it's also a classic sex position—one that never goes out of fashion. The ultimate give-and-take sexual scenario maintains its win-win qualities as one of the most popular sexercises. For the guy, it really works the shoulders and arms. Combined with the classic squat motion, it gives his glutes and thighs a great workout too. The woman will feel the benefits throughout her entire core.

MAJOR TARGETS

♂   ♀

Glutes	Spine Extensors
Deltoids	Quadriceps
Biceps	Glutes

HOT TIP

As you might expect, there is an up side and a down side to this position. The up side is obvious; the down side is that it's tricky to get into this position in the first place: The guy has to be either exceptionally strong or his partner exceptionally petite.

1 The woman kneels before a bed or an exercise bench and leans forward onto her forearms. The man stands behind her and, grasping her hips, lifts her to waist height so she can wrap her thighs around his waist.

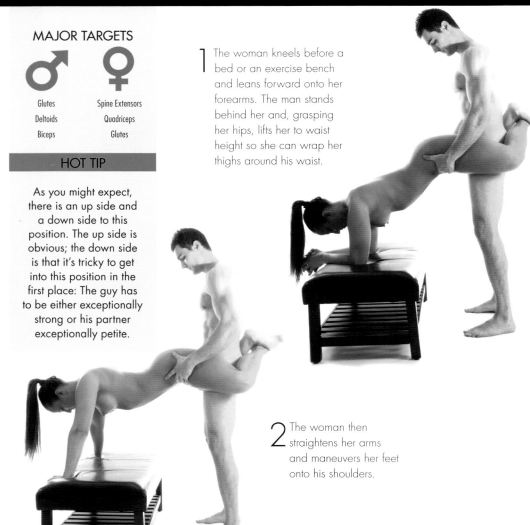

2 The woman then straightens her arms and maneuvers her feet onto his shoulders.

3 The man then bends his knees and rests his partner's thighs on his shoulders. She clasps her feet behind his head and, as he stands up, places her arms around his waist. Both partners pleasure each other orally.

4 The man then slowly bends and straightens his knees to complete a classic "squat" movement. Each partner should focus on tightening their glutes and aim to administer oral sex for three to five minutes.

HOT TIP

A man-mountain might fling his partner over his shoulder and stand like the Rock of Gibralter while she clambers into position; for most couples, however, more imagination is required—perhaps some graceful gymnastic prowess on the part of the woman, or the more prosaic assistance of a convenient bed or armchair.

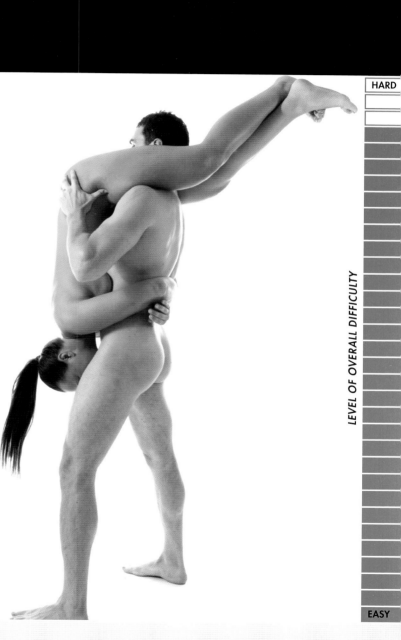

HARD

LEVEL OF OVERALL DIFFICULTY

EASY

THE CROSSROADS

This glute-sculpting sexercise offers the man a spectacular floorshow as the woman displays the full glory of gorgeous globes in perpetual motion. She enjoys the opportunity to flaunt her assets and can similarly enjoy the splendor of his chiseled pecs and abs and the lustful delight in his eyes. The wicked "you can look but don't touch" aspect of this position brings out the devil in many women and is sure to unleash the beast in her man.

MAJOR TARGETS

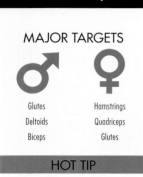

Glutes	Hamstrings
Deltoids	Quadriceps
Biceps	Glutes

HOT TIP

To make him even more horny, the woman can raise herself into a squatting position and present him with an extreme close-up of the objects of his desire. The squat position will continue to hone your glutes and tone your thighs.

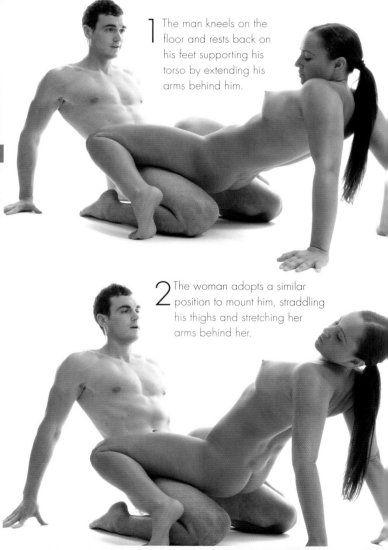

1 The man kneels on the floor and rests back on his feet supporting his torso by extending his arms behind him.

2 The woman adopts a similar position to mount him, straddling his thighs and stretching her arms behind her.

3 The lovers then focus on tightening their respective glute muscles and thrust for at least five minutes. Next, adjust the position so that the man extends his legs beneath his lover. He can then raise and lower his arms to shift the focus to his deltoids for a minute or two before returning to the original position to repeat the sexercise.

HOT TIP

The dominatrix aspect of this sexercise can drive some men crazy with lust. Once he's enjoyed the fiendish floorshow, reward yourself (and him) by standing up and, holding his hair, invite him to pleasure you orally (without moving his hands).

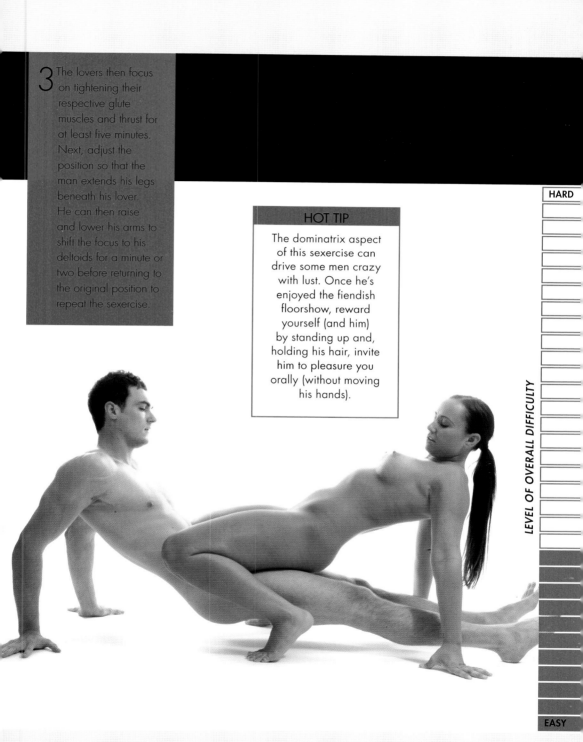

LEVEL OF OVERALL DIFFICULTY

HARD

EASY

SOLE SUPPORT

For many women, the nipples seem to have a direct sexual connection to the clitoris, and this sexercise is designed with those fortunate ladies in mind. He gets to work those neck muscles as he strains to reach her beautiful breasts with his mouth and, at first anyway, she denies access. By the time she feeds him her nipple he will know exactly what is expected of him. Meanwhile, although they will hardly notice it, both partners are getting a great glute workout.

MAJOR TARGETS

Glutes	Glutes
Hamstrings	Hamstrings
Quadriceps	Trapezius

HOT TIP

Once again, the woman is in a dominant position as the man's movement is more restricted. So she gets to dictate the action, which means going back to first base and making out big time.

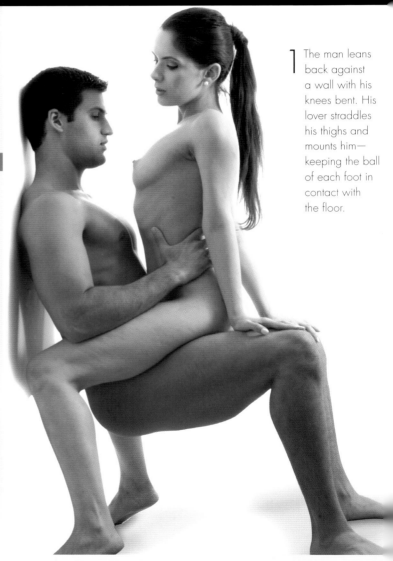

1 The man leans back against a wall with his knees bent. His lover straddles his thighs and mounts him— keeping the ball of each foot in contact with the floor.

2 Both partners clench and release the glutes as she stimulates his penis with small thrusting motions.

HOT TIP

Leaning back to show off your breast before pulling in for another necking and ear-nibbling session gives the girl a good arm and upper-back workout.

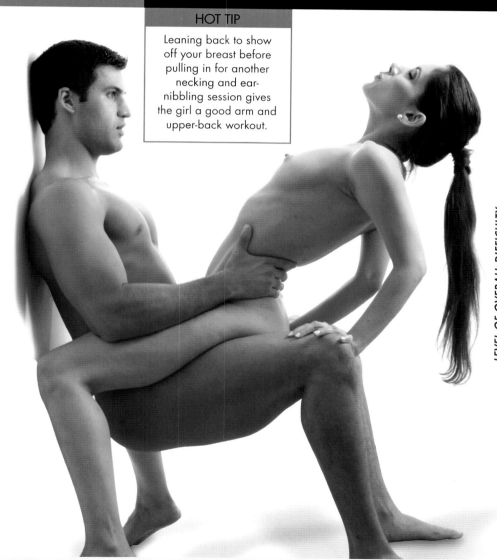

LEVEL OF OVERALL DIFFICULTY

HARD

EASY

THE SQUAT THRUST

A modification of the Kama Sutra's famous "Wife of Indrah" position, this twenty-first century remake puts Mrs Indrah well and truly in the driving seat. For dominatrix women and submissive men—or anyone who enjoys mixing things up a bit—this sexercise is hard to beat. Both partners get a great thigh and glute workout as she humps away on his penis while casually switching the remote to watch classic episodes of Sex and the City.

MAJOR TARGETS

♂ ♀

Glutes	Hamstrings
Hamstrings	Quadriceps
Pelvic Floor	Glutes

HOT TIP

Yet again, the woman is in a dominant position as the man's movement is way more restricted. The lack of eye contact heightens the impersonal aspect of this position, making it feel deliciously decadent.

1 The man lies in a supine position and raises his knees toward his shoulders. The woman place a foot on either side of his hips and mounts his penis.

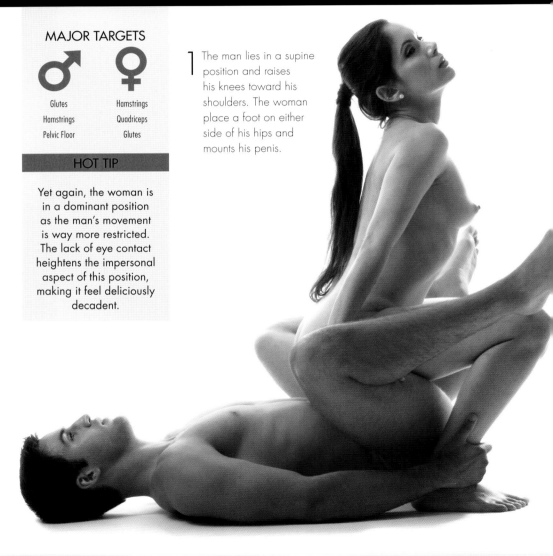

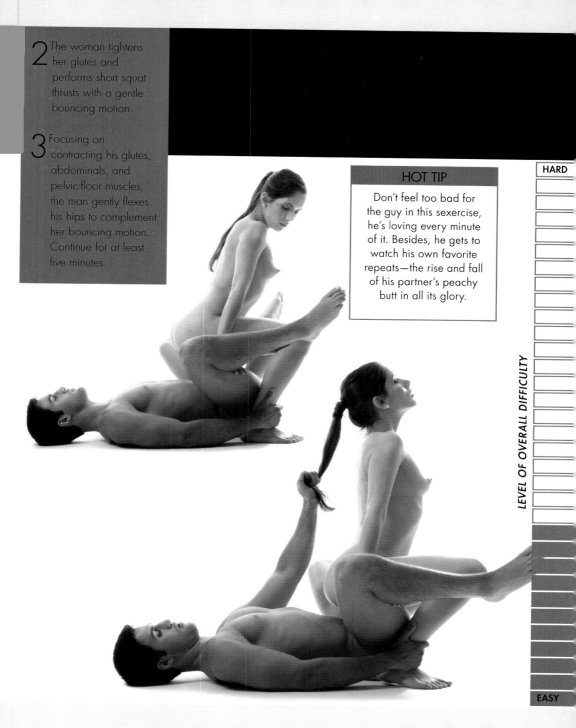

2 The woman tightens her glutes and performs short squat thrusts with a gentle bouncing motion.

3 Focusing on contracting his glutes, abdominals, and pelvic-floor muscles, the man gently flexes his hips to complement her bouncing motion. Continue for at least five minutes.

HOT TIP

Don't feel too bad for the guy in this sexercise, he's loving every minute of it. Besides, he gets to watch his own favorite repeats—the rise and fall of his partner's peachy butt in all its glory.

LEVEL OF OVERALL DIFFICULTY

HARD

EASY

GLUTES WORKOUT 1

This workout offers a range of exciting sexercises that tone the glutes and switch between male- and female-dominant postures, finishing with the ultimate expression of sexual egalitarianism—the 69 position.

BUMPING RUMPS (pages 86–87)

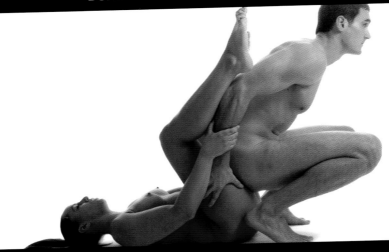

LIMBO LUST (pages 84–85)

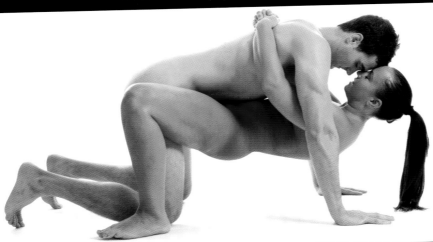

MOUNT PLEASANT
(pages 88–89)

SUMMER OF LOVE
(pages 90–91)

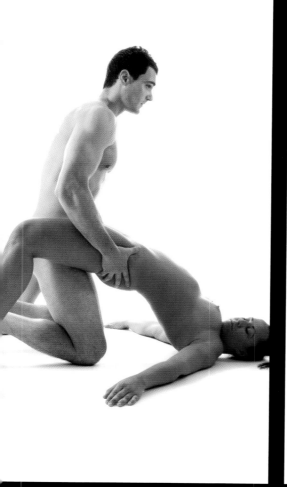

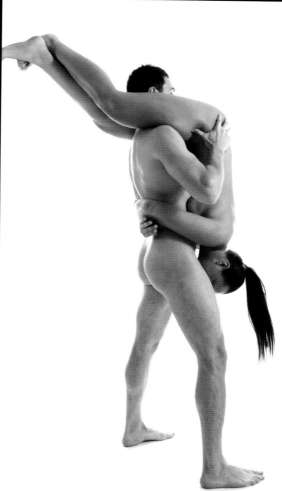

GLUTES WORKOUT 2

This workout is designed especially for the dominatrix. Feel free to spice it up with a little spanking, scratching, biting, and whatever else turns you both on.

GLUTE AWAKENING
(pages 82–83)

SOLE SUPPORT
(pages 94–95)

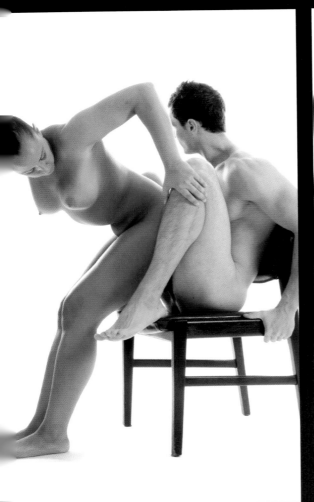

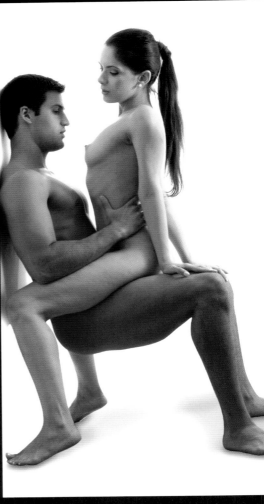

THE CROSSROADS (pages 92–93)

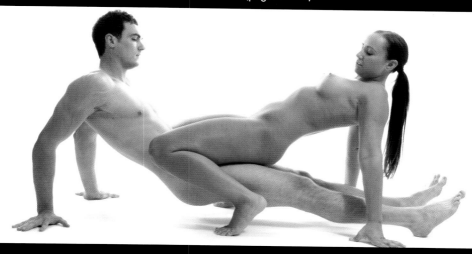

THE SQUAT THRUST (pages 96–97)

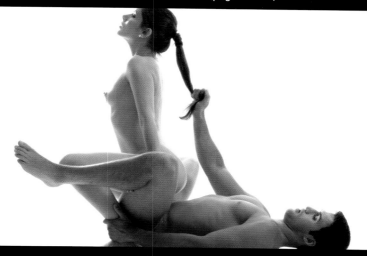

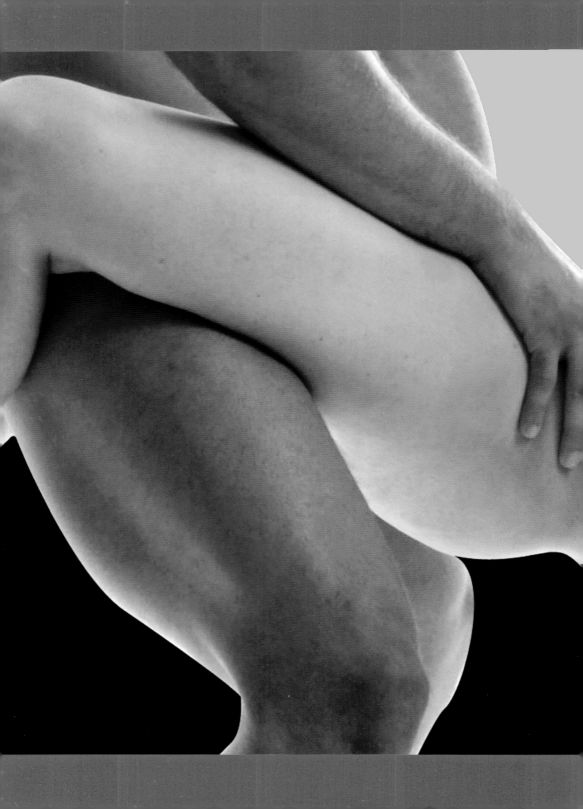

LEG SHOW

Although we can all (ladies) look great in a long evening gown—perhaps with the help of six-inch heels—when the evening draws to a close you want to be able to slip out of that gown and reveal legs that are every bit as glamorous and alluring. And, let's face it, we don't want to hide away during the summer when it's time to don those leg-baring bathing suits, shorts, and mini-skirts. Strong, toned legs also help you perform all those beach activities to the best of your ability—and even if you are lousy at volleyball, you'll still look fabulous. The main muscle groups in the legs are the quadriceps on the front of the thigh, the hamstrings at the back, and the too-often neglected inner-thigh muscles (the hip adductors) and outer-thigh muscles (the hip abductors). As far as sex goes, the latter two groups get to see a lot of action.

SKATE AWAY

For her this is a fab workout for the thighs and is especially beneficial to those oft-undervalued inner-thigh muscles. The guy works his glutes and hip flexors by thrusting from the rear, but he also works his calf muscles. He can help her to maximize the stretch by gripping her ankle and pulling gently. It should go without saying that you select Ravel's Bolero on the CD player to get in the mood for this sensual and slippery sexercise.

MAJOR TARGETS

Hip Flexors	Hip Adductors
Glutes	Quadriceps
Calf Muscles	Hamstrings

HOT TIP

If she feels like a more strenuous full-body workout, this is a great sexercise to warm up for the more acrobatic and challenging Love Lift Us Up position (see p.106).

1 The woman stands in front of the man with her back to him. Placing one hand on his waist for support, she leans forward and wraps the leg on the same side as her supporting arm around his upper thigh.

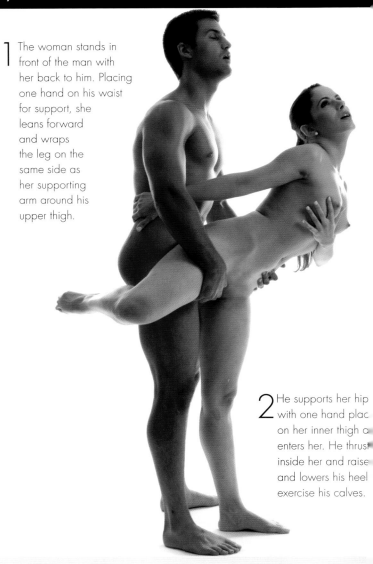

2 He supports her hip with one hand plac on her inner thigh a enters her. He thrus inside her and raise and lowers his heel exercise his calves.

3 After a minute or two she changes her supporting leg and the process is repeated. Continue alternating legs for at least ten minutes.

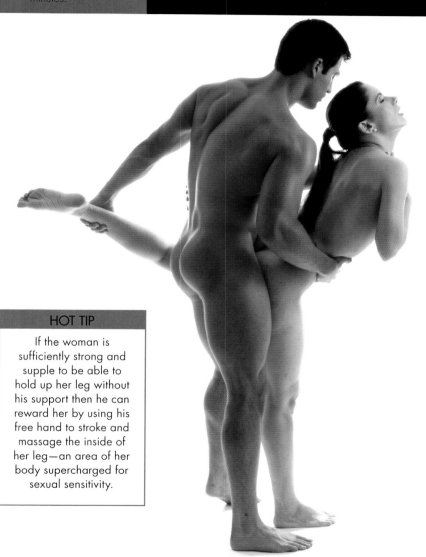

LEVEL OF OVERALL DIFFICULTY

HARD

EASY

HOT TIP

If the woman is sufficiently strong and supple to be able to hold up her leg without his support then he can reward her by using his free hand to stroke and massage the inside of her leg—an area of her body supercharged for sexual sensitivity.

LOVE LIFT US UP

Although certainly not the simplest of sexercises, this provides a great full-body workout for both partners. He'll soon feel the burn in his thighs but won't want to quit as he will feel so aroused by the psychological sense of power this sexercise gives him—not to mention the great view he gets when he glances downward to watch her glorious glutes.

MAJOR TARGETS

♂

Hamstrings
Quadriceps
Triceps

♀

Hamstrings
Abdominals
Pectorals

HOT TIP

In this position the woman can give her thighs an even better workout by alternately clasping them around his hips and then releasing them. This action can facilitate really deep penetration.

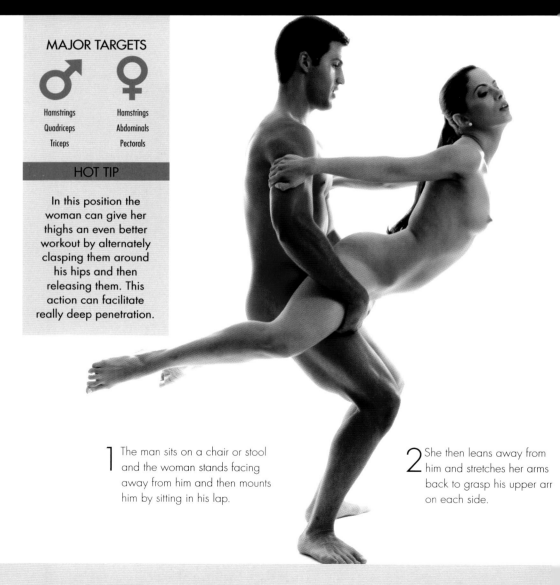

1 The man sits on a chair or stool and the woman stands facing away from him and then mounts him by sitting in his lap.

2 She then leans away from him and stretches her arms back to grasp his upper arr on each side.

3 Supporting her with his hands on her hips, the man stands up and performs squats by bending his knees until his thighs are at an angle of about ninety degrees to his lower leg.

HOT TIP

When the strain becomes too much for her, she can lower her torso toward the ground and move on to an arm and ab workout in A Matter of Thrust (see p.22) or, alternatively, she can continue to focus on her legs by reverting to the gentler Skate Away (see p.104).

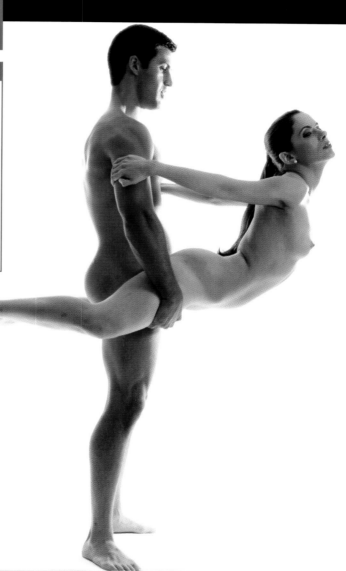

HARD

LEVEL OF OVERALL DIFFICULTY

EASY

GAMS AND HAMS

Another physically challenging sexercise, it is nevertheless extremely rewarding for both partners in terms of a physical workout and a sexual sensation. Although she appears to be very constrained in this position, she actually provides as much of the genital stimulation by using her feet as levers to raise and lower her butt.

A face-to-face position, they each get to witness the other's pleasure in their mutually lustful expressions, as she thrusts those hams and he brings home the bacon.

MAJOR TARGETS

Calf Muscles	Hamstrings
Hamstrings	Abdominals
Glutes	Deltoids

HOT TIP

Stay close to the edge of the bed and you can reward yourselves with a good cardio blast at the end of this sexercise by turning around and lowering her into the Tandem Bike position. (see p.132)

1 The woman lies on the edge of a bed and raises her legs to place them on her partner's shoulders.

2 He grasps her hips and enters her. He then clasps her forearms and pulls her toward him.

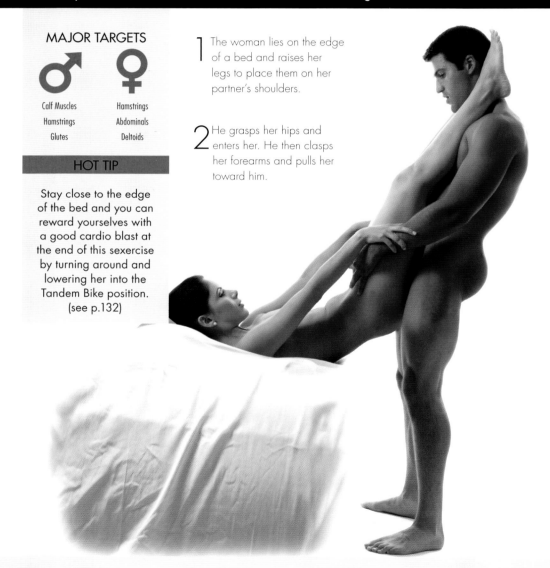

3 Grasping each other's upper arms, he then stands up straight supporting most of her weight on his legs. He then raises and lowers his heels to workout his calves, while she hooks her feet behind his head and uses the leverage to raise and lower her pelvis.

HOT TIP

An alternative finale for this sexercise is for the guy to sit down on the bed and lean back into a supine position. The woman can then squat over him and ride him into the sunset.
(see p.104).

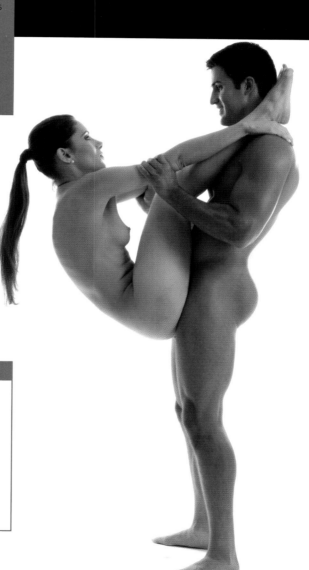

HARD

LEVEL OF OVERALL DIFFICULTY

EASY

LUSTY LIFTOFF

It really is showtime for the legs in this lusty inverted position that is not for the fainthearted. He can see nothing but her legs and she can see nothing but his butt as she grasps his powerful thighs while he bends to raise and lower her hips. The position forces the shaft of his penis downward and she will feel a powerful and highly erotic pressure against the posterior wall of her vagina as he squats over her and stimulates her with very subtle leg movements.

MAJOR TARGETS

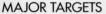

Calf Muscles	Hamstrings
Hamstrings	Abdominals
Glutes	Deltoids

HOT TIP

For guys who enjoy the occasional adventure with anal penetration (and there are plenty of straight guys who do), this is the perfect opportunity if the woman is ready and willing and happens to have a dildo and suitable lubricant conveniently to hand (as is recommended with many of these sexercises).

1 The woman lies on her back on a mat while her partner plants a foot on either side of her shoulders.

2 She then curls her legs toward her chest so that he can grasp them behind the knees and lift her up until her torso approaches a ninety-degree angle to the mat.

3 He then bends his knees to penetrate, using his quads to move her up and down on his penis.

HOT TIP

From the woman's viewpoint (and I'm talking quite literally) this is a very hardcore position. She can heighten his sexual pleasure by gently tickling his testicles or, if he finds it impossible to keep his penis inserted (as well he might), she can grasp his shaft with her hand and use it like a dildo to massage her labia and clitoris.

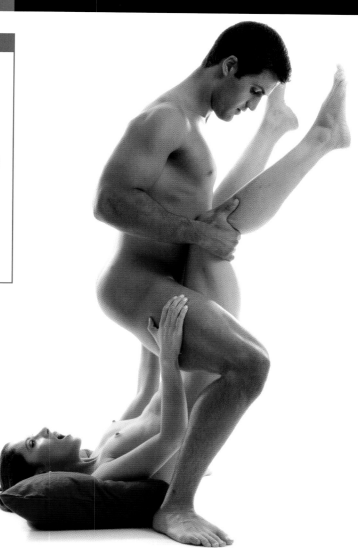

HARD

LEVEL OF OVERALL DIFFICULTY

EASY

SUMO THRUSTS

This is also known as the Battle of the Butts, although there is really no competitive element here—the man provides as much resistance as his partner is comfortable with. The guy gets to work his quads and calves while she gets a full-body workout with particular emphasis on her hamstrings. Try to keep going for three to five minutes but call time-out if you catch him picking up the *New York Times.*

MAJOR TARGETS

♂ ♀

Calf Muscles	Hamstrings
Quadriceps	Abdominals
Glutes	Deltoids

HOT TIP

Vaginal penetration is difficult in this position and, even with anal penetration, the penis is forced into an unnatural angle. He may be excited by this novel sexercise, but make sure all moves are extremely slow and steady.

1 The woman kneels down and lowers her chest toward the floor or bed and supports herself on her forearms.

2 Facing in the opposite direction to his partner, with his feet placed on either side of her, the man enters her. As she pushes steadily upward, he offers some resistance but raises his thighs to accommodate her stretch.

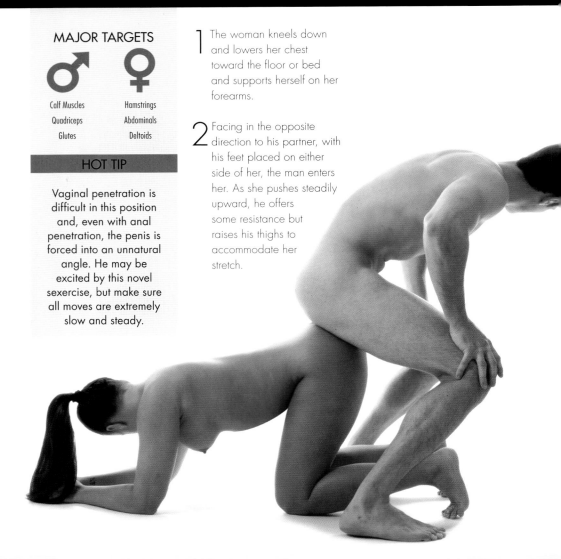

3 He then pushes gently downward as she lowers her knees to the floor. Aim to continue for five minutes.

HOT TIP

Ladies, when you first try this sexercise, you may struggle to continue for even one minute—the weight-resistance makes such a big difference. You may find it easier to push yourself up fully at the peak of the stretch, extending your legs as straight as possible. Again, just let your partner know what you are planning to do, so that he gets no unpleasant surprises that might threaten his manhood.

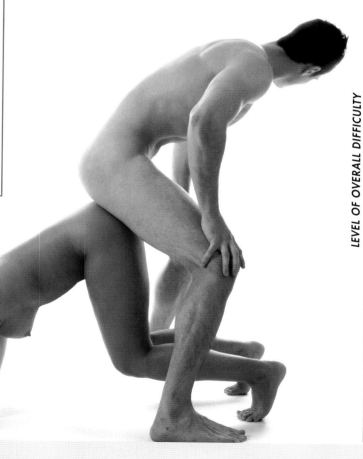

HARD

LEVEL OF OVERALL DIFFICULTY

EASY

FOR YOUR THIGHS ONLY

As the name suggests, this is a great workout for the upper leg and glutes for both partners, really targeting the quads and hamstrings. The guy is effectively in a yogic inverted bridge position, so his movement is pretty constrained. The woman does not put any weight on the guy, she is supporting her own weight and performs concentrated squats, adjusting the position of his leg (and her butt) to vary the angle of penetration.

MAJOR TARGETS

♂ | ♀
Quadriceps | Quadriceps
Hamstrings | Hamstrings
Glutes | Hip Flexors

HOT TIP

Actually, this is one for his thighs *and* eyes, ladies it's time to really show what you can do with that beautiful booty. Writhe and wiggle to drive him wild, while whittling and toning those fabulous thighs.

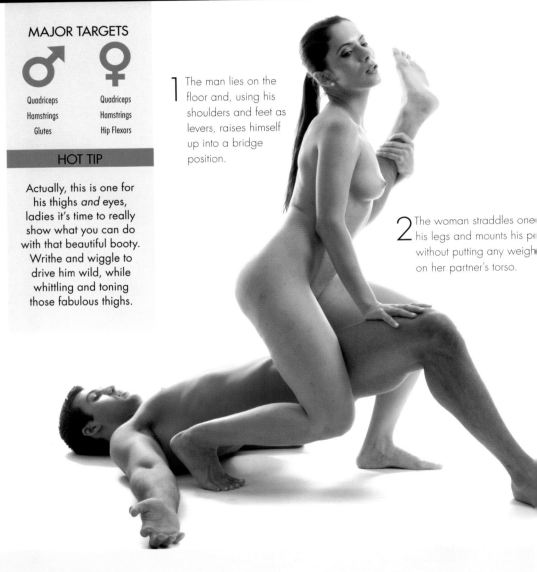

1 The man lies on the floor and, using his shoulders and feet as levers, raises himself up into a bridge position.

2 The woman straddles one his legs and mounts his pe without putting any weigh on her partner's torso.

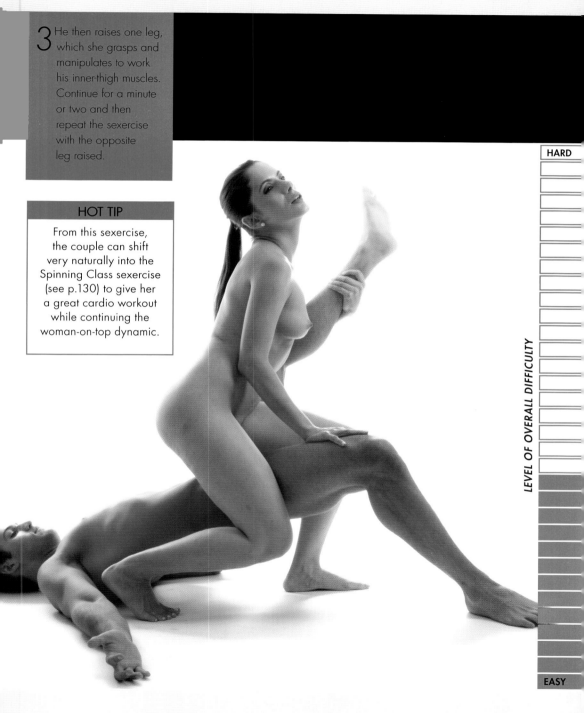

3 He then raises one leg, which she grasps and manipulates to work his inner-thigh muscles. Continue for a minute or two and then repeat the sexercise with the opposite leg raised.

HOT TIP

From this sexercise, the couple can shift very naturally into the Spinning Class sexercise (see p.130) to give her a great cardio workout while continuing the woman-on-top dynamic.

HARD

LEVEL OF OVERALL DIFFICULTY

EASY

GUESS WHO?

Straight out of the *Kama Sutra*, this is an adaptation of the classic sex position known as the Congress of the Cow. Appropriately enough, the guy gets to work his calf muscles as he raises and lowers his heels. Meanwhile, Buttercup down there gets a full workout of her own calves and thighs as she "walks" her hands slowly back and forth, mooing softly.

MAJOR TARGETS

Calf Muscles	Hamstrings
Hamstrings	Abdominals
Glutes	Deltoids

HOT TIP

Without wanting to milk the bovine analogy too much, she gets to enjoy a very horny view of his shaft penetrating very deeply in this position—provided that her udders aren't too big, of course.

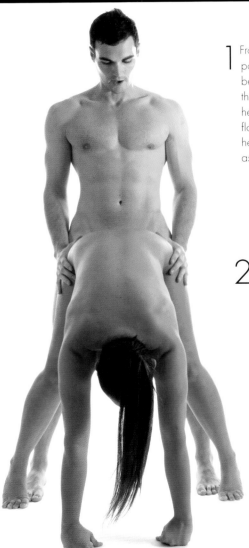

1 From a standing position, the woman bends forward from the waist and places her hands on the floor, while keeping her knees as straight as possible.

2 The man enters her from behind and commences a series of ten to twenty calf raises—flexing his ankles to raise and lower his heels.

3 Meanwhile, the woman shifts her weight to her hands and slowly "walks" them forward while keeping her legs extended, the hips up, and the back straight. Continue for at least five minutes.

HOT TIP

This is a great starting point to moove (who could resist?) into some other exciting sexercises, such as Open for Business to work the chest (see p.38) or Skate Away (see p.104) if you want to continue working your legs.

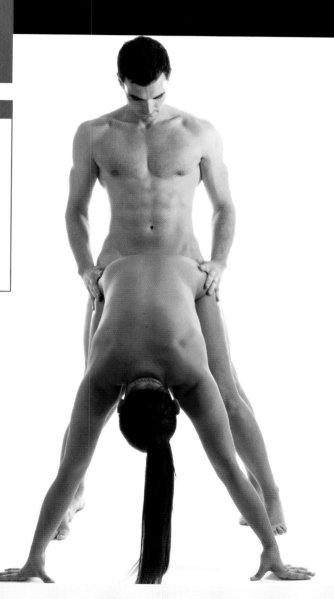

HARD

LEVEL OF OVERALL DIFFICULTY

EASY

LEGS WORKOUT 1

This workout combines four standing positions that vary in their level of difficulty. If you don't feel up to the more gymnastic sexercises, simply alternate between Skate Away and Guess Who? You'll still get a great overall leg workout.

SKATE AWAY
(pages 104–05)

LOVE LIFT US UP
(pages 106–07)

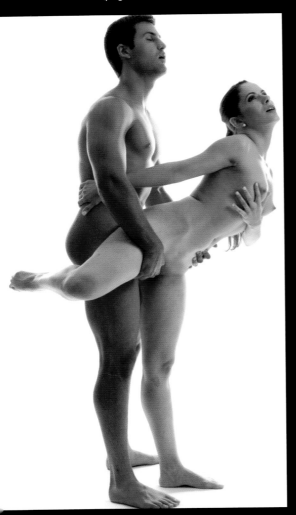

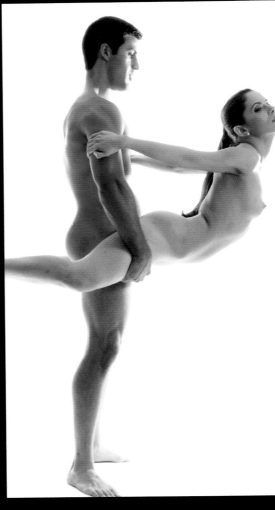

DURATION
Perform the two more challenging
position for one or two minutes, and
the others for five minutes each

SCHEDULE
Once every other week

OPEN FOR BUSINESS
(pages 38–39)

GUESS WHO?
(pages 116–17)

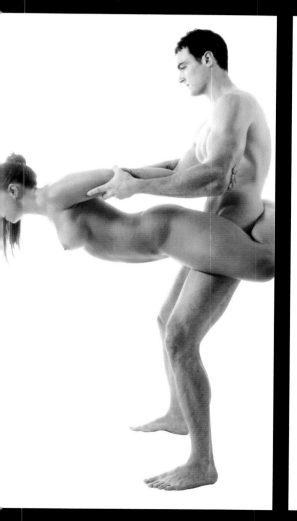

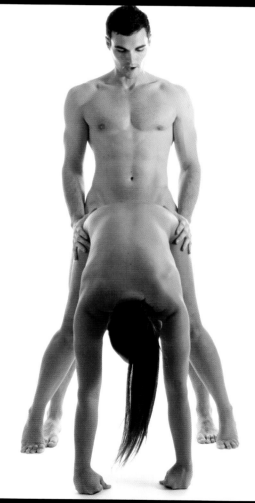

LEGS WORKOUT 2

A real mixed bag to workout those sexy stems, finishing off with a couple of sexercises where each partner gets to marvel over (or under) his or her lover's glorious glutes.

GAMS AND HAMS
(pages 108–09)

THE DIPSTICK
(pages 28–29)

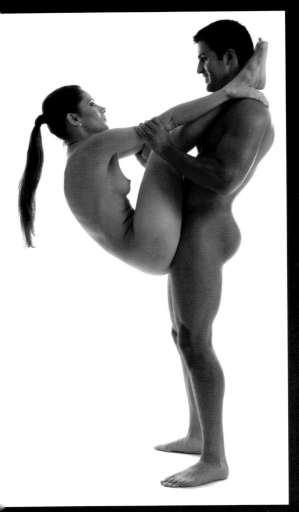

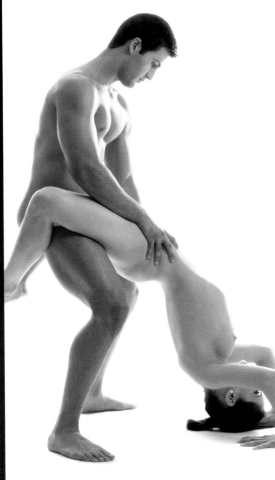

DURATION
Perform each position for
2 minutes minimum, increasing 30
seconds per additional workout

SCHEDULE
Once every other week

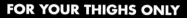

LUSTY LIFT-OFF
(pages 110–11)

FOR YOUR THIGHS ONLY
(pages 114–15)

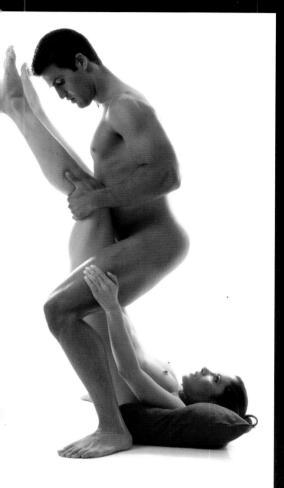

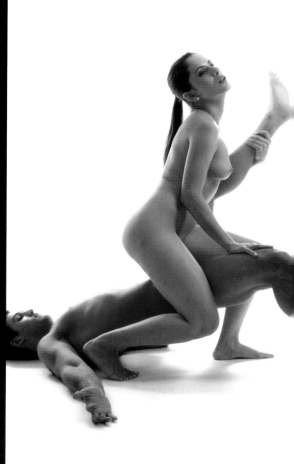

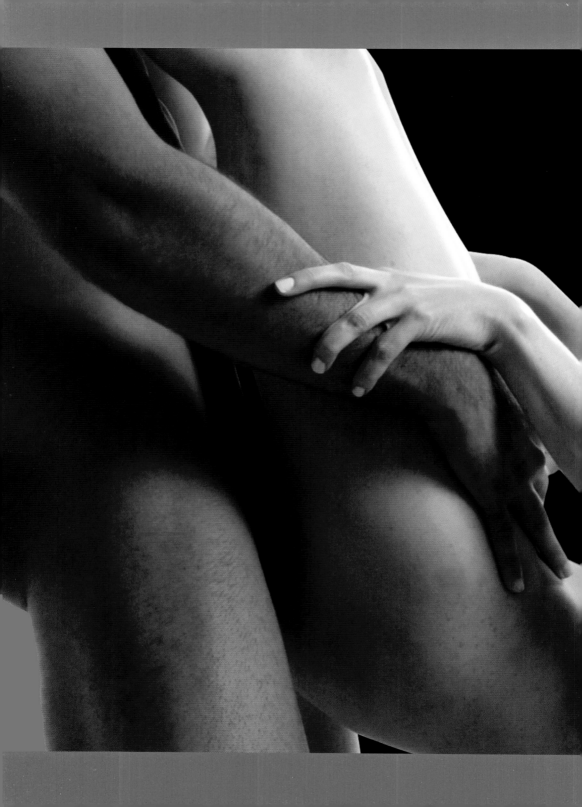

CARNAL CARDIO

Ok, it's time to get your heart pumping as well as your hips. Of course, there are few positions where you can both really go for it at the same time without doing yourselves an injury. But that's ok. The latest thinking in health terms is that the best form of cardiovascular training is "interval training," which is basically periods of intense exercise interspersed with periods of more gentle exercise—and that's exactly what we're going to do here. Many of the sexercises in this chapter allow one partner to take the reins and go hell for leather, while the other takes a well-earned rest.

Then you simply swap roles.

EROTIC AEROBICS

Erotic Aerobics is a good warm-up sexercise as she can start off at a rising trot while he engages his abdominals and soaks up the view. After five minutes you can trade places and start Bumping Rumps (see p.86), which is the male-dominant equivalent of this sexy position. But don't get too carried away here as the angle of entry is quite extreme.

MAJOR TARGETS

♂	♀
Glutes	Glutes
Hamstrings	Pelvic Floor
Quadriceps	Quadriceps

HOT TIP

It used to be thought that only women benefit from pelvic-floor exercises but they are now considered to be beneficial to both sexes—for guys, this could mean improved control over ejaculation and longer-lasting, larger erections. So, guys, get busy on those Kegel exercises. Focus, particularly, on the muscle that raises and lowers your testicles as you contract it—the same muscle that you use to control your urine flow.

1 The man lies on the floor or bed in a supine position with his legs raised and parted, and his knees bent. The woman squats between his thighs and mounts him.

2 As the man focuses on tightening his glutes and pelvic-floor muscles, the woman raises and lowers her hips in a gentle bouncing action. Continue for at least five minutes.

HOT TIP

Ladies, if you're on the edge of a bed as shown here, you can place a foot on the floor for extra stability and alter the angle of penetration to maximize your sexual pleasure.

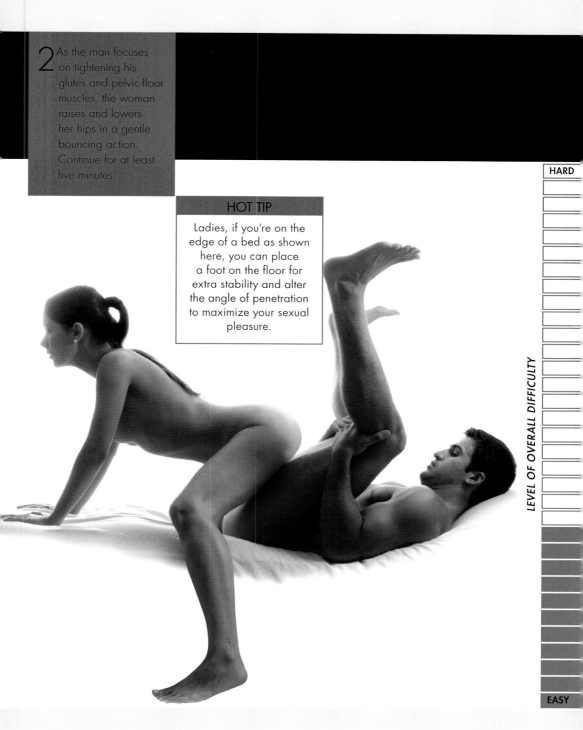

LEVEL OF OVERALL DIFFICULTY

HARD

EASY

SIDEWAYS SWING

Men who like to dominate will love this sexercise. Basically, he gets to control proceedings by "steering" her legs to one side then the other, banging away at a good pace whilst enjoying the beautiful bounce of her breasts created by his thrusting. She'll love it because the angle of penetration is constantly varied and she knows she's working on that all-important waistline as she twists ber body from one side to the other.

MAJOR TARGETS

Glutes	Hamstrings
Hip Flexors	Abdominals
Biceps	Obliques

HOT TIP

If the woman enjoys the submissive aspect of this sexercise, you can take it a step further by steering her legs upward and downward or holding them up and spreading them apart. By pushing her shins gently but firmly down toward her thighs you can both enjoy seriously deep penetration.

1 The woman lies on the bed in a supine position and raises her legs. Kneeling besdie her, the man mounts her and grasps her ankles.

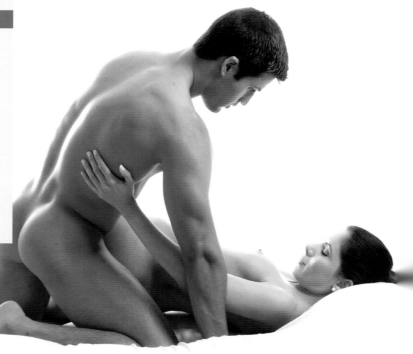

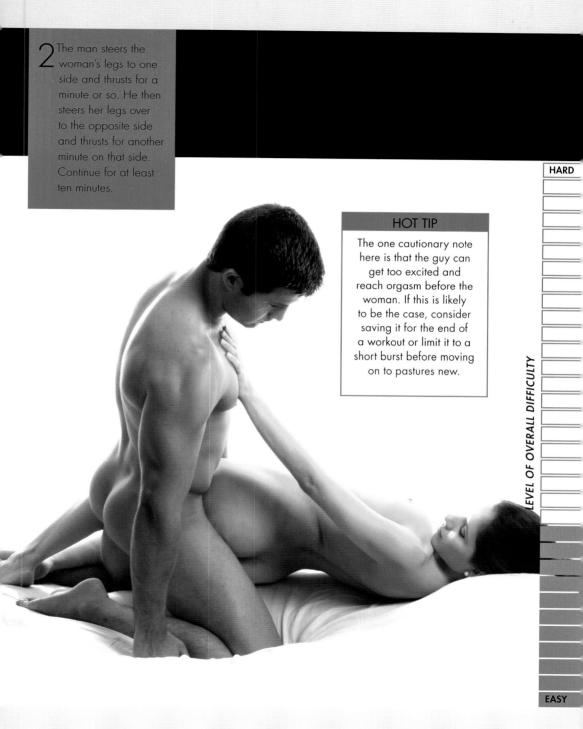

2 The man steers the woman's legs to one side and thrusts for a minute or so. He then steers her legs over to the opposite side and thrusts for another minute on that side. Continue for at least ten minutes.

HOT TIP

The one cautionary note here is that the guy can get too excited and reach orgasm before the woman. If this is likely to be the case, consider saving it for the end of a workout or limit it to a short burst before moving on to pastures new.

HARD

LEVEL OF OVERALL DIFFICULTY

EASY

DANCING IN THE DARK

After all that rough stuff in the Sideways Swing (see p.126), slow things down a little in a position that allows—no, demands—some serious smooching. You're basically simulating that classic tango step where the woman raises her knee around her partner's hip and he grasps her thigh and drags her backward with her high heels trailing. If it helps to wear heels and throw your head back occasionally, go for it.

MAJOR TARGETS

♂	♀
Calf Muscles	Calf Muscles
Hamstrings	Hamstrings
Hip Flexors	Quadriceps

HOT TIP

Each time you return to the start position, indulge in a good old necking session. And to get a good workout for the glutes, remember that you're only a few dance steps away from the Sole Support position.

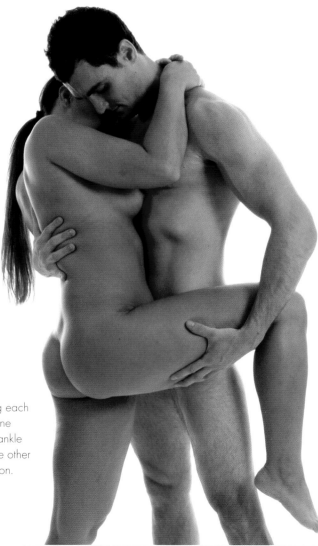

1 The lovers stand facing each other and she raises one leg, while flexing her ankle to raise her heel on the other leg, to allow penetration.

2 He takes three steps backward and then, grasping her firmly around the waist as she raises both feet off the ground, he carries her back to the starting position. She raises her other leg and the sexercise is repeated. Continue for at least five minutes.

HOT TIP

An alternative follow-on sexercise might be either the Fancy Footwork position (see p.70) where he is on top, or the Sumo Thrust position (see p.112) where she is on top. Either way, it involves a short waltz over to the bed and a quick tussle to see who ends up in the driving seat.

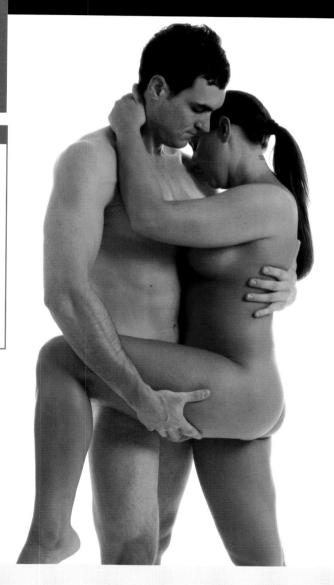

HARD

LEVEL OF OVERALL DIFFICULTY

EASY

SPINNING CLASS

After all that fancy footwork in the Dancing position (see p.128) it's time for the guy to take a well-earned rest. The Spinning Class is a classic woman-on-top position where the girl gets to hump from every angle, which means he gets to enjoy watching her from every angle. This is her opportunity to shimmy her way to fitness, putting all those hours in bellydance class to very effective use.

MAJOR TARGETS

Abdominals	Hamstrings
Hip Flexors	Abdominals
Pelvic Floor	Hip Flexors

HOT TIP

Ladies, you're getting a great workout here so don't forget your audience: When you're facing toward him, massage your breasts and tweak your nipples to drive him to distraction. When you're facing away from him, focus on shimmying those hips. (see p.94)

1 The man lies in a supine position on the bed or floor. The woman straddles his hips and mounts him in a squatting position.

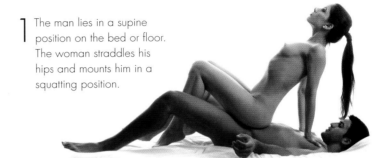

2 While the man focuses on contracting and relaxing his abdominals and pelvic-floor muscles, the woman thrusts for a minute or two before shifting around in a clockwise direction stopping at the nine o'clock position.

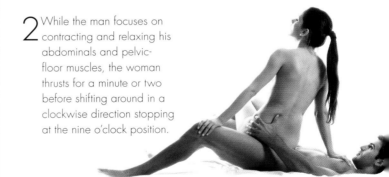

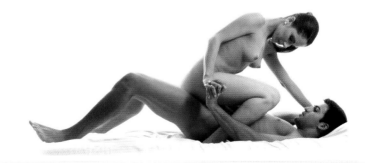

3 The woman continues to shift her position, stopping when facing directly toward her lover at the twelve o'clock position and again at the three o'clock position, before returning once more into the original squatting posture. Continue for at least ten minutes.

HOT TIP

Part of the fun here is trying to keep his penis inserted as you move around—a real challenge at times. For him, it's an opportunity to explore every part of his lover's body with his hands as well as his eyes.

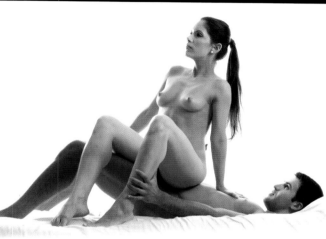

LEVEL OF OVERALL DIFFICULTY

HARD

EASY

TANDEM BIKE

If your legs are two of your finest assets then this is the one for you—the Tandem Bike allows the woman to show off the superb results of all those great workouts she has been giving her calves and thighs. For the guy, it's a chance to work his own abs and thighs, while focusing on the beauty of his lover's lean and lusty legs. Show your appreciation by caressing her calves and planting kisses on her exquisite ankles and feet.

MAJOR TARGETS

♂ ♀

Abdominals	Abdominals
Hip Flexors	Hip Flexors
Quadriceps	Quadriceps

HOT TIP

As he reclines back for the final time in his set, extend your legs luxuriously away from his chest so that his eyes can feast on those sexy stems in all their sleek and slender glory.

1 The woman lies in a supine position on a bed and raises her legs. The man kneels in front of her and she rests her feet on his chest.

2 Grasping the woman's hips, the man lifts her pelvis and enters her. She then rests her feet on his shoulders.

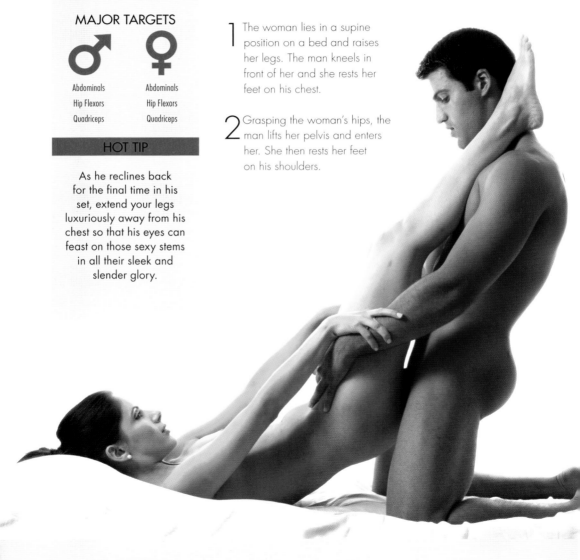

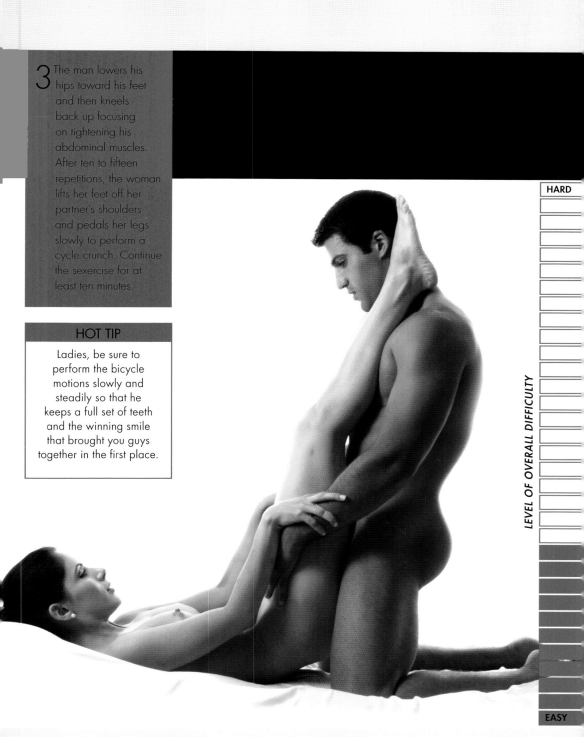

3 The man lowers his hips toward his feet and then kneels back up focusing on tightening his abdominal muscles. After ten to fifteen repetitions, the woman lifts her feet off her partner's shoulders and pedals her legs slowly to perform a cycle crunch. Continue the sexercise for at least ten minutes.

HOT TIP

Ladies, be sure to perform the bicycle motions slowly and steadily so that he keeps a full set of teeth and the winning smile that brought you guys together in the first place.

HARD

LEVEL OF OVERALL DIFFICULTY

EASY

DO THE LOTION MOTION

This feels like a very natural progression from the Tandem Bike and, in fact, the woman can continue that sexercise here by releasing her calves and pedaling away while he bumps and grinds. As well as being a great cardio workout, this is a particularly steamy sexercise that allows for lots of variation and plenty of passionate kissing.

MAJOR TARGETS

Pectorals	Hip Adductors
Triceps	Hip Flexors
Hip Flexors	Deltoids

HOT TIP

By placing his arms over the backs of her knees and leaning gently but firmly downward, the man can give her hamstrings a really good stretch. At the same time, she will be utterly constrained and vulnerable (which many men and women find very arousing) and penetration will be extremely deep and satisfying.

1 The woman lies in a supine position on the bed and raises her legs. The man kneels in front of her and leans forward to enter her, placing a little pressure on her thighs so that she can reach up to grasp her own calves or ankles.

2 He supports his weight on his arms and, while continually thrusting his hips, lowers and raises his chest toward hers to work his pectorals and triceps.

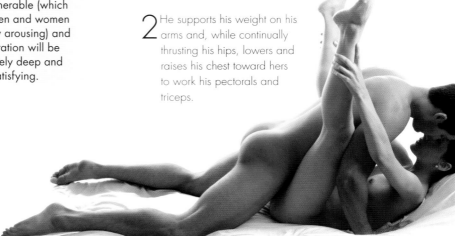

3 When the man completes a set of ten push-ups, the woman opens and closes her legs ten to fifteen times to work her inner thighs. Continue the sexercise for at least ten minutes.

HOT TIP

For fans of anal sex, this can be a particularly satisfying position. Not all anal sex needs to be rear entry and, in fact, the face-to-face position can make this the most intimate of sex acts—not just a guy wanting to dominate.

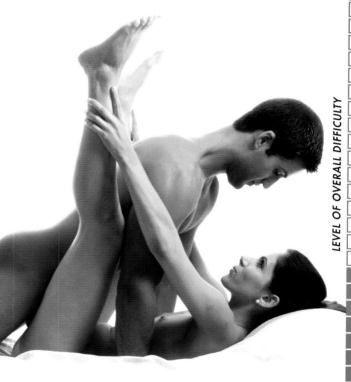

HARD

LEVEL OF OVERALL DIFFICULTY

EASY

BURN, BABY, BURN

A fabulous full-body workout and final burn, particularly for the woman's chest and arms, this sexercise can be performed on an exercise bench or the edge of a firm bed. Really go for it and get vocal, something that many couples find extremely arousing when approaching a sexual climax—although the neighbors might not be too well pleased. He, too, can encourage her vociferously and maybe even introduce a few light smacks on her butt to help her reach her goal.

MAJOR TARGETS

Pectorals	Hip Adductors
Triceps	Spine Extensors
Hip Flexors	Deltoids

HOT TIP

If she grasps him firmly enough around his waist then she can support her own weight, freeing his arms to do a bit of butt-bongo playing while singing the Mango Walk. With her permission, a little spanking might be what she needs to really enjoy this session.

1 The woman rests on her hands and knees on the edge of a bed or bench. The man approaches from behind and, holding onto her hips, lifts and enters her.

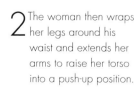

2 The woman then wraps her legs around his waist and extends her arms to raise her torso into a push-up position.

3 She aims to complete a set of eight to ten push-ups before resting down on her forearms. While she is resting on her forearms, the man performs a set of fifteen calf raises by lifting and lowering his heels.

HOT TIP

The guy can get a full leg workout here by alternating calf-raises with squats, lowering himself until his thighs are almost parallel to the floor and then standing back up again.

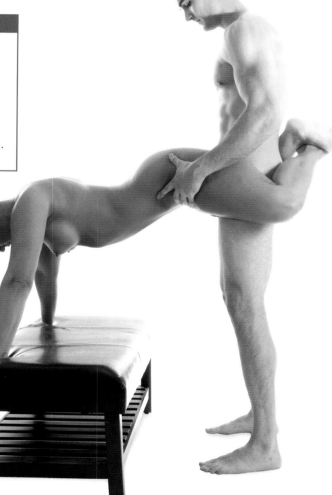

HARD

LEVEL OF OVERALL DIFFICULTY

EASY

CARDIO WORKOUT 1

This workout combines four positions that give a great cardio workout, while offering her the chance to show off those lovely legs. It starts off with a grueling pecs workout for her and, in general, this is great workout for the couple who enjoy male sexual domination.

BURN, BABY, BURN
(pages 136–37)

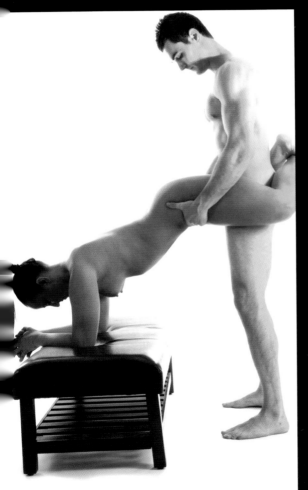

THE TANDEM BIKE
(pages 132–33)

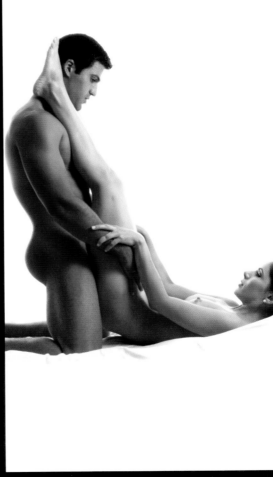

DURATION
Perform each position for 5 minutes
minimum and aim to build up to 10
minutes each

SCHEDULE
Once every week

DO THE LOTION MOTION
(pages 134–35)

SIDEWAYS SWING
(pages 126–27)

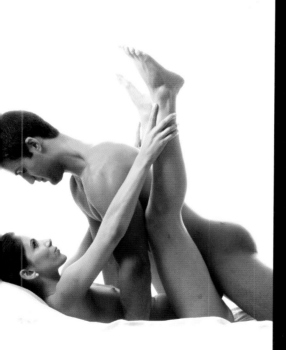

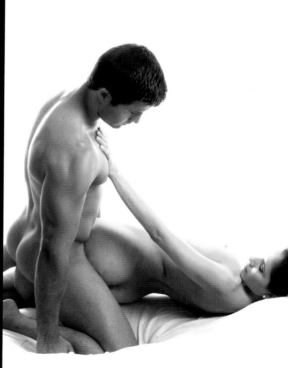

CARDIO WORKOUT 2

Here, we keep turning the tables so that both partner's get an equally thorough cardio blast. The woman comes out on top however, bringing him to an orgasmic finale with the wonderfully varied Spinning Class (see p.130).

SUMO THRUSTS
(pages 112–13)

EROTIC AEROBICS
(pages 124–25)

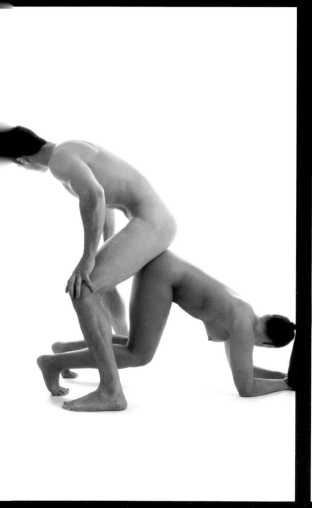

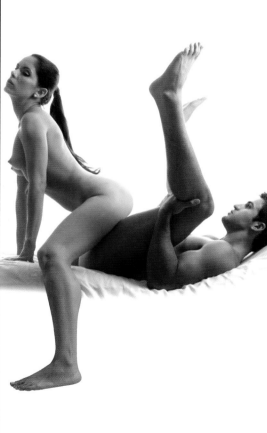

GATOR LAID (pages 44–45)

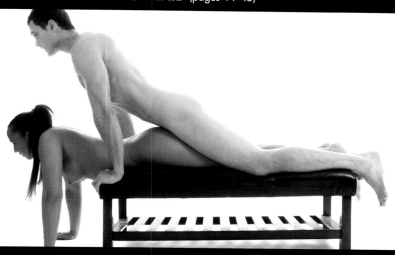

SPINNING CLASS (pages 130–31)

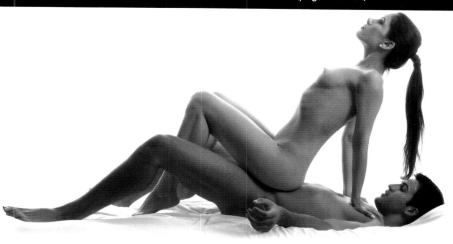

VISUAL INDEX

☐ AMOROUS ARMS   ☐ ALLURING ABS   ☐ LEG SHOW

☐ BEST CHEST   ☐ BEAUTIFUL BUTTS   ☐ CARNAL CARDIO

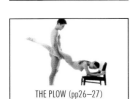

THE PULL PAIR (pp18–19)

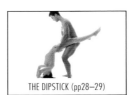

THE DIVE BOMBER (pp20–21)

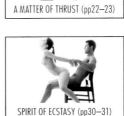

A MATTER OF THRUST (pp22–23)

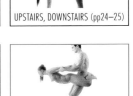

UPSTAIRS, DOWNSTAIRS (pp24–25)

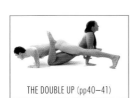

THE PLOW (pp26–27)

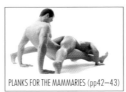

THE DIPSTICK (pp28–29)

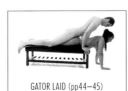

SPIRIT OF ECSTASY (pp30–31)

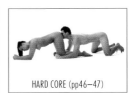

OPEN FOR BUSINESS (pp38–39)

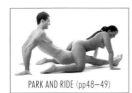

THE DOUBLE UP (pp40–41)

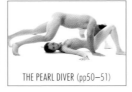

PLANKS FOR THE MAMMARIES (pp42–43)

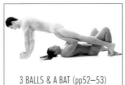

GATOR LAID (pp44–45)

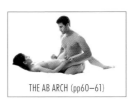

HARD CORE (pp46–47)

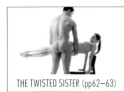

PARK AND RIDE (pp48–49)

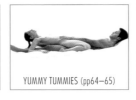

THE PEARL DIVER (pp50–51)

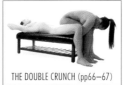

3 BALLS & A BAT (pp52–53)

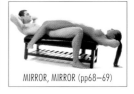

THE AB ARCH (pp60–61)

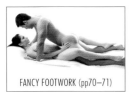

THE TWISTED SISTER (pp62–63)

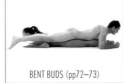

YUMMY TUMMIES (pp64–65)

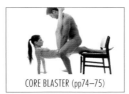

THE DOUBLE CRUNCH (pp66–67)

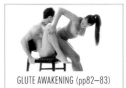

MIRROR, MIRROR (pp68–69)

FANCY FOOTWORK (pp70–71)

BENT BUDS (pp72–73)

CORE BLASTER (pp74–75)

GLUTE AWAKENING (pp82–83)